RESTORING
EMOTIONAL BALANCE
FOR YOURSELF
AND YOUR FAMILY

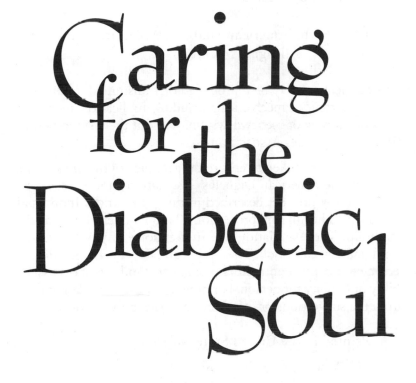

Caring for the Diabetic Soul

Foreword by Neal Friedman, MD

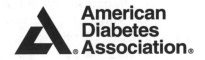

**American
Diabetes
Association**

Book Acquisitions   Susan Reynolds
Book Editor   Sherrye Landrum
Production Director   Carolyn R. Segree
Production Coordinator   Peggy M. Rote

Typesetting services by Insight Graphics
Page design by Harlowe Typography, Inc.
Cover design by Wickham & Associates, Inc.

Printed in the United States of America

American Diabetes Association
1660 Duke Street
Alexandria, VA 22314

Library of Congress Cataloging-in-Publication Data

Caring for the diabetic soul : restoring emotional balance for yourself and your family / foreword by Neal Friedman.
    p. cm.
    ISBN 0–945448–81–3 (pbk.)
    1. Diabetes--Psychological aspects. 2. Diabetics--Family relationships. I. American Diabetes Association.
RC660.4.C37 1997
362.1'96462--dc21   97–4283
                                       CIP

Editorial Advisory Board

Connie C. Crawley, RD, BS, MS
The University of Georgia Cooperative Extension Service
Athens, Georgia

John T. Devlin, MD
Maine Medical Center
Portland, Maine

Alan M. Jacobson, MD
Joslin Diabetes Center
Boston, Massachusetts

Lois Jovanovic-Peterson, MD
Sansum Medical Research Foundation
Santa Barbara, California

Carolyn Leontos, RD, CDE, MS
The University of Nevada Cooperative Extension
Las Vegas, Nevada

Peter A. Lodewick, MD
Diabetes Care Center
Birmingham, Alabama

Carol E. Malcom, BSN, CDE
Highline Community Hospital
Seattle, Washington

Wylie McNabb, EdD
The University of Chicago Center for Medical
    Education and Health Care
Chicago, Illinois

Virginia Peragallo-Dittko, RN, MA, CDE
Winthrop University Hospital
Mineola, New York

Jacqueline Siegel, RN
St. Joseph Hospital
Seattle, Washington

Tim Wysocki, PhD
Nemours Children's Center
Jacksonville, Florida

Table of Contents

Foreword

Treating the Diabetic Soul

Diabetes is not a disease that anyone wants. It usually appears unannounced and it never leaves. It is a chronic disease. If you only have experience with acute disease—one that can be cured with a trip to the hospital or by taking one round of medication—you won't know what to do with diabetes. A disease that has to become part of your everyday life requires you to change some attitudes and some behaviors. It requires you to take care of yourself in new ways. In other words, the control of diabetes depends mostly on you. Through the years, we at *Diabetes Forecast* have dedicated ourselves to helping you with self-management with articles such as the ones collected in this book. We know from people's personal histories and from many research studies that the person who achieves and keeps good control is one who accepts having diabetes and has good coping skills. You can learn coping skills.

When I think about the changes that a person needs to go through to deal with diabetes, I am reminded of the biblical prophet Jonah. Most people think of Jonah as the man who was swallowed by a whale but do not remember how he got into that situation in the first place. Jonah was commanded to travel to the great town of Nineveh "and proclaim judgment upon it." He was quite afraid because Nineveh was a large unfriendly city. He displayed classic avoidance behavior. He decided to flee to Tarshish so he would not have to accept this unpleasant task. On this journey, his ship was caught in a huge storm. His shipmates figured out that the storm was because of him and threw him overboard (much like your body may revolt if you do not control your blood sugars). Then he was swallowed by the whale. God wanted to get his attention. After three days in the belly of the whale, he decided to accept his fate and go to Nineveh. Much to his surprise, when he got to Nineveh and asked them to repent, they listened and did as he asked. Acceptance of the task and facing it head on gave him success and a lot less hassle than his avoidance behavior had done. (Likewise for the people of Nineveh.)

God spared Nineveh, which made Jonah angry. He went to the desert to sulk. He was refusing to accept again. God gave him a tree to shade him from the hot sun. Jonah remained angry, so God sent a worm to destroy the tree. Then Jonah asked to die because things were not going the way he wanted them to. God chided him for caring more about the plant than about the people of Nineveh. There is a lesson here for all of us. If you refuse to deal with the stress and anger you feel, you may destroy all the other good things that you have in your life. This is a coping skill for healthy living. All too often we focus on the small events, such as Jonah losing his shade tree and miss the big events, such as the saving of Nineveh and all who lived in it. This is a reminder to broaden your focus so you don't get stuck "not seeing the forest for the trees." Daily care of diabetes can wear you down and make you uncomfortable, but the benefit of doing it is that you can enjoy a healthier, fuller life.

I hope you will be able to use the tools in this book—no matter what age you are—to avoid making the same mistake Jonah made. Remember: the key to controlling diabetes is a healthy mind and a healthy outlook. Whenever you need to, forgive yourself, forgive others, and lighten up. Be flexible and try new ways of doing things. Don't be afraid to pick up a pencil and answer the questions you'll find in this book. The better you get to know yourself and how you do things, the easier it will be to handle your diabetes.

Neal Friedman, MD
Editor-in-Chief
Diabetes Forecast

Introduction

This is a book about parts of us that cannot be seen—our thoughts, feelings, intuitions, hopes, dreams, and fears. Living with diabetes affects and is affected by those parts of us that, although not visible, are intensely important. We cannot see the wind but we can tell the difference between a summer breeze and a hurricane. We cannot see our soul, but we can usually tell when we are out of balance, disconnected from the deepest part of ourselves. Each chapter in this book provides both questions and answers about fitting diabetes into our lives, work, family, and our inner selves. The questions and the answers herein are opportunities to pause and reflect on what is uniquely true for each of us. An answer that works for one person will not suit another. A question that is profoundly meaningful to one of us will not resonate with another. This is a book about caring for the diabetic soul, our souls, your soul.

The chapters in this book were originally articles in *Diabetes Forecast*. In some ways they go together like a symphony. The same themes are revisited but by different instruments. When journeying to the heart and soul of living with diabetes, we need to peer into the center of one's being through the different windows provided by different chapters. Many of the chapters focus on similar issues, such as who am I, what is most important to me, how can I live the life I want with diabetes, what can I learn about myself and the world from dealing with my diabetes? However, each of these chapters addresses these issues from a different perspective. Some chapters may appeal to you more than others. Also, a chapter that does not seem meaningful today may be very meaningful a year from now. Like a complex piece of music, this book is meant to be experienced over and over again. Because, as we change, the message and the impact of these chapters will change as well. Think of this as a book of meditations, a mirror that can reflect some aspect of the soul of a person with diabetes—a soul that must be cared for if we are to live life to its fullest.

R.M. Anderson, EdD

Part I:
Nobody's Perfect

1
Denial?
(Not Me!)

by Marilyn Rollins

Most people deny the diagnosis of diabetes when they first hear it. "I don't believe it," "It can't be true," or "You must be mistaken," are common responses.

That first denial is not likely to cause problems. In fact, it's so common that some physicians think it may be part of the acceptance process.

Continued denial, however, is quite another thing. It prevents you from gathering the knowledge and developing the skills, discipline, and attitude necessary for accepting responsibility for your own health.

Why Deny?

Denying the seriousness of diabetes or the necessity for following all of your diabetes

3

care instructions is tempting. Denial allows you to ignore your daily health care plan. It enables you to lower your standards for good health.

Your denial gives your family permission to minimize your health care needs, too. People who love you—your mother, father, sister, brother, husband, or wife—may want to help you feel better about your life, or save you from the work necessary for good care. They may simply find your diabetes difficult to deal with.

Whatever the reason, your denial allows them, as well as you, to avoid facing the fact that diabetes is a lifelong, chronic illness, which, if untreated, may have serious consequences.

Subtle Denial

Denial that occurs at the time of diagnosis is obvious and fairly easy to deal with. The forms of denial that happen later are more subtle and much more difficult to recognize.

What's more, people with diabetes and their families are not the only ones who indulge in denial. Even some medical professionals may occasionally fall into this trap. That's why it is so important for you, the person with the disease, to pick up the clues of denial. You must be on your guard and not interpret someone else's denial as permission to slight your diabetes regimen.

You can rationalize neglecting almost any part of your health care, including the need to take insulin or medications, lose weight, stop smoking, exercise regularly, or lower cholesterol. It's also easy to deny other aspects of care such as the necessity to monitor your blood glucose levels, maintain professional foot and eye care, and consult with other health care professionals at appropriate times. Just because denial is so pervasive, however, doesn't mean it's easy to spot.

Spotting the Denial

Certain phrases can help you flag denial. Occasionally a medical professional who does not specialize in diabetes care may talk about a borderline or mild case of diabetes, or say there is "just a touch of sugar" in your blood, or that you should "watch your sugar intake."

Though well-meaning, these terms send the wrong message. They deny the simple fact that anyone who has consistently high blood glucose readings has diabetes.

And here are some things you may tell yourself to keep diabetes at arm's length.

* I can skip it this once.
* I'll do better next time.
* One bite won't hurt.
* This sore will heal by itself.
* I won't go to the doctor until...
* I don't have time to...
* My insurance doesn't cover...
* My diabetes isn't serious. I only have to take a pill, not "shots."

Such statements keep denial alive.

Mega-Denial. Although denial can reach into every aspect of diabetes care, there is one area where almost everyone practices mega-denial, and that is diet.

All of us like the foods we've enjoyed all our lives. And many of us are used to three full meals a day in addition to morning and afternoon snacks, TV munching, and, perhaps, midnight refrigerator raids. To change either the times or the foods we eat is no easy task.

That's why, when a doctor advises someone with diabetes to see a dietitian, follow a meal plan, and change his or her eating habits, the result is often denial. It takes many forms, but here are a few of the most common:

* It's too expensive to see a registered dietitian.
* I'm a meat and potatoes man.
* So-and-so has diabetes and she eats whatever she wants.
* I don't like "rabbit food."
* My family won't want to change what they eat and I don't want to eat alone.
* There's no place to buy healthy food where I work.
* It's too hard to bring my lunch.
* I've tried, but I just can't change what I eat.

If your eating plan consists only of avoiding sugary foods or following a printed diet sheet, you are denying the fact that you need a detailed, personalized, up-to-date food plan.

Dangerous Denials. Blood glucose self-monitoring is yet another area that invites denial. Self-monitoring can provide vital knowledge to help you keep your diabetes in control, but regular testing can be a nuisance. So you may decide that you "know" what your blood sugar is by how you feel.

However, "knowledge" of blood glucose levels based on feelings can be incorrect. It can lead you to overeat or undereat or exercise inappropriately. It can even mislead others into thinking all is well with you when it is not.

If you haven't been testing regularly, you might review your testing technique with a certified diabetes educator. Also, you might let your family and friends know your monitoring schedule so they can encourage you.

It's also easy to deny the need for foot care. Washing and checking your feet daily is part of a good diabetes health care plan, whether you have insulin-dependent (type 1) or non-insulin-dependent (type 2) diabetes. It's important to wear low-heeled, well-fitting, comfortable footwear.

But you may find foot care too time consuming, or you may like the style of a pair of shoes—even if they rub your feet. So you say, "This sore will heal by itself" or "I can't run to the doctor with every stubbed toe." Convenience, money, or fashion may be your excuse to deny the fact that you could be courting foot problems.

If you have type 2 diabetes and make remarks such as, "I don't need to take my medications every day—after all, it's not like I'm on insulin," then, whether you realize it or not, you are practicing denial.

You may even deny the need to stop smoking or chewing tobacco. Nicotine use by someone with diabetes can contribute to a number of complications affecting their kidneys, eyes, heart, and brain. Yet people find ways to deny that the amount of nicotine they use is harmful. "I only take a few puffs," "I only smoke when I'm nervous," and "It keeps me from eating too much" are common expressions that mask denial.

Since the possibility of getting complications is a difficult subject to face, it is clearly one that's ripe for denial.

After all, it is comforting to say that future problems "will never happen to me" or that there will be a cure before long, so "I don't need to take care of myself now."

All denials are potentially dangerous because any denial allows you to sabotage your own health care.

Avoiding Denial. One way to avoid denial is to state or write down clearly your specific diabetes care instructions and your health care goals. It's important to realize that it will take time to reach those goals. Don't expect to change your habits—especially eating habits—overnight.

Be firm, even aggressive, about your diabetes care. Encourage your family and friends to help, and let them know that being indulgent with you is not a kindness.

It can actually lull you into thinking everything is all right, causing you to end up with lower-quality health care.

Ask your certified diabetes educator for help if you are denying some aspect of your diabetes. Consult a registered dietitian for help with a food plan, especially if you are still denying the need to eat well some years after diagnosis.

Review your medications with your physician routinely, and schedule annual appointments with an eye doctor who understands diabetic retinopathy. Let your dentist know that you have diabetes before you undergo examinations, dental surgery, or even general dental work.

If your denial is due to exhaustion from following the same plan day after day, year after year, review your food plan and diabetes regimen with an appropriate professional to see what changes can be made.

In short, accept the diagnosis of diabetes. Recognize the forms that denial takes. Understand that controlling diabetes requires daily attention, and take the responsibility for that attention.

Additional Payoffs

Sure, it takes a certain amount of bravery to recognize and confront denial. But those who do confront it reap great benefits—and not only in terms of health.

When you say no to denial, you are saying yes to health. You may also find that your self-esteem is enhanced by your refusal to hide from an unpleasant reality. The more honestly and openly you deal with diabetes, the more you retain control.

Marilyn Rollins, RD, CDE, *is a nutrition consultant in private practice in Phoenix, Arizona. She is a published author and past president of the ADA Arizona Affiliate.*

2

Feel Good About You

The way you feel about your diabetes can affect the way you feel about yourself.

by Sandra Schwartz

Aristotle, one of the world's great philosophers, offered an invaluable bit of advice to his students: Know thyself.

If he were alive today, he might add: And know how you feel about having diabetes. He'd probably agree with today's scientists, who are finding that the more you come to terms with having diabetes (whether it's insulin-dependent [type 1] or noninsulin-dependent [type 2]), the better you feel about yourself.

So how do you really feel about having diabetes?

Not an easy question. After all, it's hard, and sometimes painful, to look inside yourself. But this three-part quiz may help. (Of course, such a general do-it-yourself exercise is not intended to replace the services of a mental health professional, especially if you are having problems coping with the emotional side of diabetes.)

I. How You Feel About Yourself

You are the one who determines what to eat, how much to exercise, and when to test.

* How often do you "pretend" you don't have diabetes by ignoring details of diet, insulin or medication, testing, or exercise?

0	1	2	3	4	5
Often		Sometimes			Never

* How often do you feel angry about something either directly related to your diabetes, or to your life in general?

0	1	2	3	4	5
Often		Sometimes			Never

* How often do you feel depressed about something either directly related to your diabetes, or to your life in general?

0	1	2	3	4	5
Often		Sometimes			Never

* How often does your diabetes seem to interfere with other aspects of your life, such as work, school, family, or friends?

0	1	2	3	4	5
Often		Sometimes			Never

If your score in the "How You Feel About Yourself" category is 10 or more, you are probably aware of what's going on inside your head. What's more, you generally like what you find there.

But if your score here is less than 10, look again. Some of your feelings about diabetes may be hidden, even from you. Worse, without you realizing it, they may be keeping you from having a positive view of yourself.

Although it's easy to deny diabetes when it comes to the daily regimen (who hasn't skipped a blood glucose test or eaten something not on the food plan?), it's far more difficult to deny it inside.

That's why surface denial can lead to feelings of guilt. But unfortunately, you may not understand what the guilt is all about, so you continue dealing with your diabetes in the same way.

Where does that leave you? With still more guilt.

When this kind of pattern develops, you can wind up with a negative self-image that makes you angry and depressed. And that anger and depression can last so long, and be so well disguised, that you might not realize that it's rooted in your struggle to accept diabetes.

Anger can surface in unsuspected ways, too. For instance, you might find yourself overreacting to a friend's innocent remark. Something like, "You never want to go out anymore," may provoke you to start an argument, a reaction that might surprise even you.

Anger or depression may also be the reason you decide that co-workers don't like you, or that you don't look good in your clothes anymore.

What to do?

Realize that before you can begin to feel better, you have to become aware of what's really going on. Try to focus—honestly—on how you feel about having diabetes. Does it make you angry? Are you fighting diabetes at every turn?

Try to separate your emotional responses to the disease from your responses to other aspects of your life.

Then deal with those feelings directly involved with diabetes. If necessary, ask for professional help.

II. How You Feel About Others

* How many of your friends, family, and co-workers have you told about your diabetes?

0	1	2	3	4	5
None		Some			Many

* How many of your family and friends do you feel comfortable with discussing your diabetes?

0	1	2	3	4	5
None		Some			Many

* How many of your family and friends have accurate information about diabetes?

0	1	2	3	4	5
None		Some			Many

* How many of your family and friends are sensitive to your diabetes needs?

0	1	2	3	4	5
None		Some			Many

Your answers to this section can help you see how you relate to others where diabetes is concerned. If your score here is 10 or more, your diabetes is probably not interfering with your relationships.

But once again, if your score is less than 10, take another look at how you interact with others.

That doesn't mean that you must tell everyone you meet that you have diabetes. Nobody expects that. But if you keep your diabetes a secret from people who are close to you—say, a romantic interest or close friend—you may discover that you are actually having trouble accepting it yourself.

You'll probably also learn that keeping a secret, and fearing its discovery, has unseen consequences.

Secrets can affect a relationship in subtle, negative ways.

When you withhold important information, it makes it hard to be close to others in many ways. And when the fact that you have diabetes finally does come out—as it most likely will—the idea that you kept it a secret will probably be far more important to the other person than the diabetes itself.

Of course, it's true that some people who know that you have this disease may "get in your way" about it. They think they are experts and don't hesitate to tell you exactly what you should do to take care of yourself.

But if you get angry, and then keep that to yourself, too, you're doing yourself another disservice. Keeping diabetes a secret, or ignoring remarks that annoy you, can distance you from others.

Worse, these reactions can affect the way you see yourself. Keeping a secret can make you feel disloyal. And not responding to people's remarks can make you feel inadequate and put down.

Instead, try to decide which people in your life deserve to know that you have this disease. Then find an appropriate way to tell them.

Next, try telling those who are overbearing or misinformed about diabetes that you don't welcome their remarks. You might add that their advice is inaccurate, if it is, and explain what they have wrong. Finally, let them know you are handling things just fine, thank you.

Diabetes can be a lonely and isolating disease even in the best of circumstances. Allowing it to make you submissive, or bottling up your feelings, pushes you even further away from potential friendships.

Letting those you care about know you have diabetes while keeping its control in your own hands may spark a change, not just in how others act toward you, but in how you feel about yourself.

Diabetes can be a lonely and isolating disease.

III. How Are You Handling Your Diabetes?

* I am comfortable with the many aspects of my diabetes care.

   0   1   2   3   4   5
   Never   Sometimes   Often

* I accept the fact that I must spend time on my diabetes care.

   0   1   2   3   4   5
   Never   Sometimes   Often

* I am successful in managing my diabetes care.

   0   1   2   3   4   5
   Never   Sometimes   Often

* I integrate diabetes into my life.

   0   1   2   3   4   5
   Never   Sometimes   Often

This section can help you scan your feelings about the repetitive, daily requirements of diabetes care. If your score here is 10 or more, that part of your life is probably going well.

But if you score less than 10, it's possible that you seriously resent the time that diabetes care takes from your day.

Such resentment is not unusual. After all, integrating good diabetes management into a busy, active life is difficult at best.

And even though your friends may also incorporate a healthy diet or a regular exercise program into their lives, their need to do so is not as pressing as yours. They have more choice in the matter.

But the truth is, you have choices, too. You are the one who chooses how to manage your diabetes from hour to hour, day to day. You are the one who determines what to eat, how much to exercise, and when to test.

If you can accept this fact for what it is—control—you can take a giant step toward feeling good about yourself.

Aristotle may not have been correct about everything he said, but his "know thyself" was right on target.

It's the beginning of a healthy, exciting spiral. First you know yourself, then you know and accept your diabetes. That helps you feel better about yourself, which, in turn, helps you gain even better control over your disease. And you know where that leads: feeling better about yourself.

Sandra Schwartz, MHS, *is a diabetes counselor at the Eleanor and Joseph Kosow Diagnostic and Treatment Center of the Diabetes Research Institute in Miami, Florida. Schwartz has had type 1 diabetes since childhood.*

3

Controlling Your Stress

by Pauline Fisher

Your boss just told you that the project you worked on for three weeks has to be redone. * The radio announcer just reported a major backup on the highway. * Your mother-in-law (whose only concession to low-fat cooking is substituting margarine for butter in all her specialties, and whose after-dinner conversations consist solely of "Have some dessert—just this once") is coming to visit tomorrow—for 2 weeks...

Stress is a part of life. But chronic stress wears you down—physically, emotionally, and spiritually. Stress can also affect your diabetes control. Hormones released during stressful periods may cause the levels of glucose and fatty acids in your blood to rise. Certain stress hormones can decrease insulin release in people with type 2 diabetes.

You have little control over the traffic, and even less over your mother-in-law's cooking, but you do have control over how you react to stressful situations. Deep breathing relaxations, body movement and awareness activities, and feeling/thinking checks will start you on your way to a less stressful life. Here's how to start.

Breathing Relaxations

Sit in a chair or lie on the floor, uncross your arms and legs, and relax. Take a very deep breath through your nose, filling your body with as much air as you can. When you exhale, empty out as much breath as you can. Inhale deeply again, and as you exhale, feel the breath wash through your body from your head all the way down and out your feet. Repeat again and feel the tension loosen, melt away, and leave your body. Once more as you breathe in, smile inwardly, feeling a relaxed quality washing over you.

As you repeat the process, follow your breath from body part to body part down your body. Feel it first enter your lungs, then the rest of your body down to your toes.

If thoughts enter your mind, take note, and let them wash away with the next breath. Do not get attached to your thoughts. Bring your attention back to your breathing—in and out, in and out. When you are ready, bring your attention to how your body is making contact with the chair, or floor if you are lying down. Open your eyes, feeling refreshed and relaxed.

Breathing exercises can be done from 5 to 20 minutes at a time. Set aside one to three specific times a day to do these. It is important for you to give yourself permission to stop what you are doing and relax. Even if you have to go into a bathroom and lock yourself in for a few minutes—take the time.

Once you have practiced these exercises and feel comfortable with them, try doing them at a moment when you feel stressed or overwhelmed. Love yourself enough to care.

Move, Dance, Be Aware

Your body must be free before your mind can function to its fullest extent. By circling, stretching, and shaking, you can loosen and articulate your joints and your whole body and feel awakened and more alive.

Start with your head. Rotate it slowly a few times in both directions. After a few circles, you may quicken the pace if you'd like. Continue the process of circling, moving down the body, part by part—shoulders, wrists, arms, rib cage (if you can), torso, hips, legs, and ankles.

When you have completed circling, begin again at the top of your body and move down, stretching each body part in all directions. Be creative. Think of your body like a twisty or a pipe cleaner making unusual shapes. Feel like a cat, tuning in to your body. Stretch where your body wants you to stretch.

When you have completed stretching, shake out each and every part of your body, concluding with a whole body shake. Now you will feel completely invigorated.

You can do this body-freeing exercise with or without music, inside or outside, sitting for parts of it or standing and moving around.

If you are using music, you may want to use one piece for stretching and another for shaking.

Dance. Another fun body-part warm-up and loosening activity is to do a dance with each part of your body. Again, find music that appeals to you. Beginning at the top of your body, do a dance with your head, moving it in time to the music or to your own rhythm. Enjoy investigating different ways to move your head as well as exploring the many ways it can move through space (up, down, back, and under).

When you've finished the head dance, move down to your other body parts and do a dance with each until you feel that you have greased all your joints. At this point, you'll begin feeling warmer and looser; you will have brought more oxygen into your lungs and increased your blood circulation.

Category Dances. Another playful and fun way to warm up and loosen your body is Category Dances. One of my favorite categories is Sports, because it requires active and full body requirements. Pick some movements from sports—for example, pitching, batting, running, and sliding from baseball; kicking, running, throwing, and catching from football; and dribbling and shooting from basketball. Select some music, put all of these movements together, and do them as a full-out dance to the music.

Feeling/Thinking Check

Your perceptions, your thoughts, and the things you choose to focus on all affect your feelings, and your feelings affect your thoughts. You are responsible for your thoughts: You can choose your responses.

"I'll never get good control of my diabetes" after just one poor test result, or "That mistake I made cost us the whole project" are thoughts that wear you down, and they don't solve anything.

Begin to take note of your thoughts. If you start to feel anxious, trace your thoughts for the last half hour. Soon, you'll realize more quickly when a negative mood has started. It may take some effort for this to become habit, but the rewards will be worth it when you realize that you can and do have control over yourself.

To stop negative thoughts, put a rubber band on your wrist. Each time you become aware of obsessive, worrisome, or negative thoughts, gently snap the rubber band. Eventually, you may not need the rubber band—you'll be able to say "stop" to yourself and go on to other thoughts. You can also "reframe": replace the bad thought with a better thought. Or try thinking of a favorite poem, prayer, uplifting quote, or positive mental image.

Use the Tools

These are a few tools for managing stress. But none of these will work if you leave them, forgotten, in a tool box. Learning stress-reduction techniques, but not practicing them regularly and integrating them into your daily life, is like learning physical exercises and doing them once a month or only when your body feels unfit, tight, or overweight.

Stress is part of life, and each of us has to take responsibility for our responses to it. So begin a new habit.

Find the tools you can commit to, then use them. Just start.

Pauline P. Fisher, MA, *teaches stress management at the Center on Aging, University of Maryland, College Park. She is founder of A Moving Experience, an organization dedicated to creative stress management and movement awareness in Washington, D.C. She conducts workshops and training seminars around the country and is the author of* Creative Movement for Older Adults: Exercises for the Fit to Frail *(Human Sciences Press) and* "The Relaxation & Imagery Tape."

4

Beyond the Blues

by Lee Schwartz

Feeling down occasionally is normal. Feeling depressed for more than a couple of weeks is not.

Your mood may change from day to day, or even hour to hour, as bad and good things happen at home, work, or school. This is normal.

But sometimes your mood bottoms out and stays there. Life seems hopeless. That's depression, and it needs to be treated.

Simply having diabetes doesn't necessarily make you more prone to depression than people who don't have the disease. But the stress of daily diabetes management may aggravate a bad situation and open the door to depression.

Diabetes management means carefully monitoring your blood sugars. It means following a special diet and taking insulin shots or other medicine for diabetes all the time. You may feel all alone or different because of all the special work you do in order to live with diabetes.

If you develop complications, or if you aren't able to keep your blood glucose as near normal as you or your doctor would like, you may feel like you're losing control over your diabetes. Even tension between you and your doctor may make you feel frustrated and sad.

Any of these experiences can bring on the blues. But when the sadness just won't go away, day or night, for two weeks or more, that might be a sign that you're developing a serious problem.

Unfortunately, many depressed people don't ask for help. They think their bad feelings will just go away, or believe that they can't be helped. For a person with diabetes, this can be especially bad. If you are depressed and have no energy, you will hardly be able to carry out regular blood sugar monitoring. If you feel so anxious that you can't think straight, it will be hard to keep up with a good diet. Or you many not eat at all. These situations can play havoc with your blood sugar levels. It's actually very basic: Recognizing depression is vital to good diabetes management.

When to Get Help

If you have been feeling really sad, blue, or down in the dumps, see if you have any of these symptoms:

* You've lost interest or pleasure in previously enjoyable activities.
* Your sleep patterns have changed: You have difficulty falling asleep, you awaken frequently during the night, or you want to sleep more than usual, including during the day.
* You wake up early in the morning (between four and six) and aren't able to get back to sleep.

* Your appetite has increased or decreased, with corresponding weight gain or loss over a relatively short period of time.
* You have difficulty concentrating. For example, you aren't able to watch a TV program or read an entire newspaper article because other thoughts or feelings get in the way.
* You have less energy than usual; you feel washed out all the time.
* You feel nervous all the time and can't sit still because of anxiety.
* You are less interested in sex.
* You cry frequently.
* You feel guilty about things you've done, or feel that you're a burden to others.
* You feel worse in the morning than during the rest of the day.
* You feel like you want to die, or you're thinking about ways to hurt yourself.

If you have three or more of these symptoms, or if you have just one or two symptoms but you've been feeling bad for two or more weeks, it's time to get help.

Tell your doctor about your symptoms. He or she will first look for possible physical causes for your depression. For example, too much alcohol drinking or drug use can contribute to feelings of depression. A person who drinks to avoid feeling down can end up feeling more depressed.

Sometimes people take tranquilizers in high doses or over long periods of time to deal with anxiety. But this also can bring on, or deepen, depression.

Other prescription drugs, including medications for high blood pressure and pills for Parkinson's disease, can cause depression in some people. This does not mean you should stop taking your medicine, but do discuss any side effects with your doctor.

If you do have symptoms of depression, don't wait too long to get help.

Other possible physical causes of a depressed mood include: disorders of the thyroid; too little or too much of certain electrolytes (sodium, potassium, chloride) in the blood; vitamin B_{12} or folic acid deficiency; or the anemia that comes with these vitamin deficiencies.

You should be aware that poorly managed diabetes can cause symptoms that look like depression. During the day, low blood sugar (hypoglycemia), from too much insulin or other diabetes medication, may make you feel tired or anxious. Hypoglycemia can lead to hunger and overeating. If you have hypoglycemia at night, your sleep may be fitful or interrupted by awakenings, or if, instead, your blood sugar is high, you may get up frequently at night to urinate and then be tired during the day.

Again, if you are experiencing any of the symptoms of depression, don't keep it to yourself. See your doctor.

Call in a Specialist

If your depression is not caused by something your regular doctor can treat, he or she should refer you to a specialist. You might consult with a psychiatrist, psychologist, psychiatric nurse, psychiatric social worker, or a certified or licensed professional counselor.

All of these mental health professionals can guide you through the rough waters of depression, but if medications are called for, a psychiatrist (a medical doctor with special training in diagnosing and treating emotional disorders), must be consulted either by you or your mental health provider. Only a psychiatrist can prescribe medication and treat the possible physical causes of depression along with the psychological causes.

Depression and the Elderly

Mrs. F., a widow of 72, who had had diabetes for many years, came to see me 18 months after she had suffered a stroke. Despite the gains she had made since her recovery, Mrs. F. seldom left her house. Yet even as she cried, telling me how different she felt, how different she thought she appeared to others, and how unattractive she felt, she said she was not depressed.

Mrs. F.'s depression and her reaction to it are not unique. Depression is the most common psychiatric problem doctors find in older people. As many as 20 to 35 percent of elderly people with medical problems become depressed. Older persons, in particular, may become depressed after the loss of a family member or friend. Yet many don't go for help.

If you are an older person with diabetes, you may feel depressed over your inability to function on your own because of diabetes complications. If you have just learned you have diabetes, you may become depressed because of all the new responsibilities that come with living with diabetes.

Unfortunately, you may not be willing to say, "I feel depressed." Maybe you're afraid that needing help for intense depression means being thought of as "crazy."

You might not even feel "depressed." Instead, you might find yourself complaining that you feel really nervous, or that you can't concentrate or remember things. You may complain of aches and pains or problems in your body instead of a problem with depression.

It's important to recognize depression and get treatment. Fortunately, Mrs. F.'s daughter encouraged her to seek help. Mrs. F. learned that depression can be treated, even when the illness that preceded the depression—such as a stroke or diabetes—will remain.

To simplify a very complicated matter, there are two tracks of treatment for depression. One is psychotherapy, the other, antidepressant drugs; many people benefit from some combination of these two approaches.

Psychotherapy with a well-trained therapist with whom you feel comfortable can help you examine the problems that bring on depression. Most therapists use one or more of the following approaches:

Insight-oriented (talking) therapy is an ongoing conversation between you and your therapist, exploring your thoughts and feelings in order to resolve the sad feelings.

Usually the process involves comparisons of how you interact with people (including the therapist) today as opposed to how you related to significant people in your past. The goal is to allow you to live today without being hampered by the past.

Supportive therapy aims to restore an earlier and healthier way of functioning. This therapy, which also consists of talking, may help you discover ways you dealt with stress in the past. It helps you apply what you've learned to help you function today.

Cognitive therapy for depression is a time-limited treatment aimed at correcting negative thoughts about yourself and your negative view of life and the future. Cognitive therapists try to teach you to change the assumptions upon which your negative thoughts are based. Cognitive therapists try to instill new beliefs that do not lead to feelings of depression.

Brief psychotherapy is a short-term use of talking therapy to change or stop the problem and produce a more positive adjustment to life. Brief psychodynamic psychotherapy lasts about 10 to 20 sessions and looks for a connection between current problems and past experiences. It requires high motivation because it brings out strong emotions.

Social therapies analyze those persons or groups (affiliations) that you have available to provide understanding and reassurance. This could involve marital or even family therapy.

You may need help to repair relationships. Sometimes, you may do or say things that push others away when you need their help the most. You may not even be aware that you are doing this. Therapy with you and your significant others aims to help all of you find better ways to support each other.

Depression itself can hinder your search for help. Your support networks may have fallen away over time, leaving you isolated. A mental health professional can help you to build new networks. For severe depression, supports may include day hospitals, day treatment programs, or other community programs, which help you develop better relationships.

If you feel alone because of your diabetes, depression can develop or get worse. A diabetes support group can be very helpful. For older adults, adult day care or support groups can help. For children, diabetes camp can provide a wonderful social experience.

Medications

Sometimes, depression can't be treated by psychotherapy alone. In this case, you may need to take medications for your depression. Doctors prescribe antidepressants when they suspect that the depression they are treating is caused by an abnormality in the chemistry of the brain. Antidepressants are medications that help restore normal brain chemistry.

It takes from three to four weeks for an antidepressant to boost your mood. But certain drugs will help you from the start, by helping you sleep or by allaying anxiety.

Antidepressants

Here are some commonly prescribed antidepressants and some of the side effects you may experience:

* Heterocyclic antidepressants may lower blood glucose in people with diabetes, so make sure your regular doctor or diabetes care team are involved in deciding whether or not you should be pre-scribed these drugs.

  Heterocyclic antidepressants include imipramine (Tofranil), nortriptyline (Pamelor, Aventyl), and desipramine (Norpramin). Nortriptyline and desipramine are less likely to cause side effects such as dry mouth, constipation, or dizziness than other hetero-cyclic antidepressants. Nortriptyline, imipramine, amitriptyline (Elavil), and doxepin (Sinequan, Adapin) may cause sleepiness and decreased anxiety, so these can be good choices for someone who is not able to sleep or relax. Heterocyclic antidepressants may affect your heart, so if you have had heart problems, your regular doctor should be consulted before you take these drugs. Also, some people gain weight while on these drugs. This may be a side effect or simply the result of the improved appetite that comes from recovery from depression.

* Newer agents like trazodone (Desyrel), fluoxetine (Prozac), ser-traline (Zoloft), and paroxetine (Paxil) seldom cause dry mouth or constipation, but trazodone can lower blood pressure, and fluoxetine, sertraline, and paroxetine can cause anxiety or sleep-lessness at the beginning of treatment.

  Fluoxetine, sertraline, and paroxetine sometimes cause gas-trointestinal discomfort, but these problems can usually be avoided by taking the medication with food. Fluoxetine may affect blood sugar control. It sometimes lowers blood sugar, espe-cially if you use insulin or an oral agent, and sometimes high blood sugar occurs when the medicine is stopped. If you take this drug, consult your doctor if your blood sugars begin to fluctuate.

* Monoamine oxidase (MAO) inhibitors, like phenelzine (Nardil) or tranylcypromine (Parnate), while safe and effective when used appropriately, are used less often because they require a special diet. In addition to diabetes requirements, you would have to avoid cheeses, certain wines, and other foods, as well as many over-the-counter drugs, or serious high blood pressure can result. Low blood sugar, though rare with MAO inhibitors, is more likely when a heterocyclic antidepressant is given along with an MAO inhibitor.
* Less commonly used medications include lithium carbonate and the tranquilizer alprazolam (Xanax).

Sometimes lithium or thyroid medicine is added to a heterocyclic antidepressant to help the antidepressant work more effectively.

Make sure you tell your therapist and the consulting psychiatrist about your diabetes and any other health conditions you have. Sometimes antidepressant medication can affect your blood sugar and may have other side effects (see "Antidepressants," on page 30). In most cases, the changes in blood sugar control can be managed by changing, with your doctor's advice, your dose of insulin or other diabetes medication.

All medications, including antidepressants, have side effects, but medications are prescribed whenever the benefits outnumber the possible side effects. The best way to know what to expect is to discuss your medication fully with the doctor who is treating you. Don't let the possibility of side effects deter you from taking antidepressants. If you don't take antidepressants when they are needed, you are leaving untreated a very treatable, and serious, illness.

Recovery

If you do have symptoms of depression, don't wait too long to get help. And if your doctor can't refer you to a mental health professional, contact your local psychiatric society or the psychiatry department of a university medical school, or the local branch of organizations for psychiatric social workers, psychiatric nurses, or mental health counselors. Your local affiliate or chapter of the American Diabetes Association may be able to help you find a mental health professional who has worked with people who have diabetes.

If it's important to you that insurance cover part of the cost of treatment, check with your insurance company beforehand. Many insurance plans have very specific conditions relating to referrals to a psychiatrist or other mental health professional that must be met for the treatment to be covered.

Recovering from depression gives you the opportunity to move forward. Living will seem easier again as symptoms are treated. You'll also be better able to cope with diabetes. You will feel more in control, and being in control brings you the chance to exercise choice about how you want to live your life.

Remember, depression can be treated. If you need help, get help.

Lee S. Schwartz, MD, *a clinical associate professor of psychiatry and behavioral sciences at Northwestern University Medical School, is in private practice in Chicago.*

5

Get Your Head Ready for Exercise

Dreading the start of your new exercise program? You're not alone. Here are six common hurdles—and ways to leap them in a single bound.

by Harold J. May

Face it. We like things easy. That's why there's fast food, self-cleaning ovens, and remote control channel changers.

Exercise just doesn't fit the bill. It's hard and it's time-consuming, we tell ourselves. All sweat and discomfort.

Then the internal dialogue begins: How do I start? Where do I start? I've got too much weight to lose! I just don't know if I can do it.

That's about as far as some folks get before they collapse back into the cushions. Don't be one of them. Negative thoughts are roadblocks, sapping your will at every turn. Here are six tips to help you overcome them.

1. Stop the Debate!

George succeeded in starting a morning walking program. But then...hmmm...his legs seemed sore, and...hey!...then his back did, too. Every morning when he woke up, he looked out the window to see if it was raining. He looked for any excuse not to go.

George hadn't yet made a real commitment to an exercise program. His constant debate, the back-and-forth thoughts about whether or not to exercise, made exercise seem like a tremendous chore.

Once George decided that, no matter what, he would take his morning walk, his internal debate ended. Then exercise wasn't a burden, it was simply something he did—period.

If you have not yet made a firm decision to exercise on a regular basis, take time and think it through again. It may not be an easy decision, but it will be easier if you choose not to debate it over and over again.

When you make a firm decision to begin, your new lifestyle will unfold more easily.

2. Set Realistic Goals

After watching the recent Olympics, Mary felt that she wanted to be like those well-conditioned athletes that we all saw on TV. Then she immediately gave up any thought of exercising at all, knowing she could never reach that goal.

If your goals are set too high, you're sabotaging yourself. You need to set reasonable goals. The goals should also be reachable in a reasonable amount of time.

For example, a goal of dropping two dress sizes by your daughter's wedding three months from now may not be the best goal for you. For one thing, you probably shouldn't drop that much weight so quickly. For another, the goal is too far away. You'll be tempted to work hard to lose weight in the beginning and again near the end of the three months, as your deadline looms.

You'll do better if you don't set a weight-loss target. Instead, set daily goals in terms of small distances or the number of minutes you'll walk or exercise. Then, gradually increase those as you become more comfortable with your exercise program. Establish the habit and the enjoyment first; weight loss will follow.

3. Enlist Allies

Americans typically pride themselves on being self-reliant, independent, and strong-willed. Consequently, many people try to begin an exercise program by toughing it out alone without the support of others.

Some people don't even tell others that they're trying to exercise. They want to surprise people with their great new shape. They feel that if they tell people, others will know if they fail, or that family members will nag them when they take a day off from exercising.

This is not starting smart. People who actively arrange a support system for their exercise efforts are more likely to succeed.

When you decide to start exercising, ask for the support you'll need. You'll want an ally at home and at work.

Enlist a family member or close friend to walk with you in the morning. Join an athletic club together.

Form a neighborhood exercise club so that you and several friends can exercise together each week on a regular basis.

Ask your family to give you praise and rewards for your efforts. Ask them not to remind you of past difficulties or failures. Nagging or attempts to police you won't work, either. Ask them to point out positive changes (such as improved mood and energy) that they see also.

4. Look for Early Changes

Harriet noticed soreness in her muscles after two weeks of an aerobics class. But instead of seeing this as a negative, she began thinking that these were muscles that were now being used and were becoming stronger.

Exercise stimulates the body in many positive ways: It rejuvenates your blood's supply of oxygen and releases mood-elevating chemicals to your brain. You can quickly begin seeing exercise as a pick-me-up rather than something to be dreaded or avoided.

Focus on the positive. Notice your increased energy level. Pay attention to your increased lung capacity and breathing abilities. You may notice an improvement in your blood glucose levels, even within the first week of your exercise program.

5. Keep the Habit Through Thick and Thin

Beginning an exercise program is like establishing any habit. It takes a conscious effort to make it succeed, and you need to do it every day to get the new habit firmly established.

Each of us encounters daily temptations to put off exercising. It's easy to say, I can do it tomorrow, I don't have time to do it today, I don't have anyone to go with me. If you give in one day, it's easier to give in the next...and the next. You've got to keep the habit—even if you don't make your goal that day.

Before You Start

Although most people with diabetes can exercise safely, exercise involves some risks. To shift the benefit-to-risk ratio in your favor, take these precautions:

* Have a medical exam before you begin your exercise program, including an exercise test with EKG monitoring, especially if you have cardiovascular disease, you are over 35, you have high blood pressure or elevated cholesterol levels, you smoke, or you have a family history of heart disease.
* Discuss with your doctor any unusual symptoms that you experience during or after exercise such as discomfort in your chest, neck, jaw, or arms; nausea, dizziness, fainting, or excessive shortness of breath; or short-term changes in vision.
* If you have diabetes-related complications, check with your health care team about special precautions. Consider exercising in a medically supervised program, at least initially, if you have peripheral vascular disease, retinopathy, autonomic neuropathy, or kidney problems.
* Learn how to prevent and treat low blood glucose levels (hypoglycemia). If you take oral agents or insulin, monitor your blood glucose levels before, during, and after exercise.
* If you have type 1, and your blood glucose is above 250 milligrams per deciliter, check your urine for ketones. Don't exercise if ketones are present, because exercise will increase your risk of ketoacidosis and coma.
* Always warm up and cool down.
* Don't exercise outdoors when the weather is too hot and humid or too cold.
* Pay special attention to proper footwear. Inspect your feet daily, and always after you exercise.

Let's say you and a co-worker have decided to walk for a half-hour Monday through Friday at 3 p.m. You both stick with it for four days. Then on Friday at 2:30, your boss declares a crisis. You're looking at two hours of frantic labor. You absolutely, positively can't take a half-hour break.

OK, accepted. But you've got to keep the habit. You and your exercise partner should change into your walking shoes, walk outside, then come right back in and go back to work. Don't even have time for that? Then change into your walking shoes, keep them on for 10 seconds, then change out of them and go back to work. You didn't exercise, but at least you didn't break your new, still-fragile habit. You're still on track for next week. When 3 p.m. rolls around, you'll be reaching for your walking shoes like you reach for your toothbrush every morning.

When you stick with a plan for at least one month, you're well on your way to establishing an exercise habit, one that can be long-lasting and enjoyable.

6. Thinking Makes It So

The human mind has the power to create feelings out of thin air. For example, you can create hunger just by thinking about your favorite meal.

You can use this power of the mind to maintain your exercise program.

Foster an "exercise self-image." Every morning for a month say to yourself, I am a person who exercises. You'll soon believe it. And this new self-image will have a powerful effect on your behavior.

When you think of yourself as someone who exercises regularly, you will behave as someone who exercises regularly. You'll be able to view exercise and physical activity as something positive and a part of you rather than something negative or something you are forced to do.

Lastly, keep life's hassles in perspective. Perhaps you have known people who get very upset with the least little mishap and others who handle a crisis without falling apart. Your ability to "roll with the punches" will be particularly important during your first few weeks of exercising. The key to maintaining perspective on life's hassles is the realization that the way you think about a situation will determine your feelings about it.

Begin to think of exercise as a chance to improve your health and enjoy the experience at the same time. Thinking really does make it so.

Harold J. May, PhD, *is associate professor of Family Medicine and section head of Behavioral Medicine at East Carolina University School of Medicine, Greenville, North Carolina.*

6

Forbidden Thoughts

by Cynthia Herbert Adams

The more you try not to think about fat-laden goodies, the more you will.

Close your eyes. Now, DON'T imagine a pink polka-dotted elephant sipping from a straw. Whoops. I think I know what happened. You just imagined a pink polka-dotted elephant sipping from a straw. That's exactly what happens when someone tells you not to think about cakes, candies, or french fries. And that's why some people with diabetes—children as well as adults—become obsessed with food.

Foods and Diabetes

Eating appropriate foods—and not eating inappropriate ones—is so much a part of both insulin-dependent (type 1) and non-insulin-dependent (type 2) diabetes treatment that having the disease almost forces you to focus on diet. Usually, that means focusing on what you are not going to eat. "I won't have the chocolate cake at Nancy's party," "I won't have ice cream at the beach," or "I won't order steak at the restaurant tonight."

But the more you deny yourself certain foods, the more you tend to think about them. It's the pink polka-dot elephant problem.

Although most people with diabetes learn to turn their attention away from food, some continue to concentrate on it. That thinking and rethinking becomes a form of self-hypnosis; eventually it turns into an obsession.

Be Positive

Food obsessions can happen to anyone who has to cut food items from the menu. Yet everyone in that predicament doesn't become food obsessed.

One reason is that different people may approach food restrictions in different ways. The ones who do best take a positive approach to the new dietary restrictions. Instead of dwelling on what they won't be eating, they look forward to what they will be eating at the next meal or snack.

They also look for substitutes for their favorite treats, and that's never been easier to do than now. Stores today offer a wide variety of commercially prepared foods for people on a low-fat or low-sugar diet. (Of course, it's still necessary to read the nutrition facts to make sure each product is truly low in fat or sugar.)

A growing number of food labels also list exchanges according to the American Diabetes Association and The American Dietetic Association's *Exchange Lists for Meal Planning.* That, too, makes it easier than ever to work a treat into your food plan.

Room for Favorites

There are still other ways to make healthy food choices without totally restricting your menu.

Food plans list the number of calories, carbohydrates, proteins, and exchanges for one day—not one meal. By planning the day's menu carefully, you may be able to include something special.

The American Diabetes Association and other health organizations recommend that we get no more than 30 percent of our calories from fat. That recommendation, too, is for the entire day. Again, it is possible to arrange a day's menu to include a slice of cake at a party (perhaps with a minimum of frosting) or a piece of steak at dinner, if the rest of the day's calorie percentages take that extra delectable serving into account.

Remember, too, that an exercise program, approved by your physician, may allow for special snacks once in a while.

Best Way Out

However, the most productive way to stop thinking about food is to make people and activities, not food, the focus of your life.

It should not surprise anyone that people who have many non-food interests are usually physically and mentally healthier than those who focus mainly on what they are going to eat. The non-food people are also likely to stick closer to their diabetes regimen.

On the other hand, the more a person feels restricted, the greater the danger that he or she will become bitter and angry. Among people with diabetes, that can lead to eating items not on the food plan—and doing it often. Clearly, how you handle food restrictions makes a difference.

The "No-No" Voice

Some people with food restrictions make the mistake of cultivating an inner police officer. Such a constant "no-no" voice means they are always being reminded of what they can't have, which almost guarantees that they'll defy the voice eventually.

Then, after the voice has "made" them eat chocolate cake, it usually tells them how "bad" they were. That creates a desperate desire to be "good." So they promise themselves that all eating will stop for now, which starts the cycle all over again.

Binging and Starving

The binge-starve cycle is not unusual, but it is extraordinarily dangerous for anyone with either type of diabetes. Binging and starving will destroy an insulin-management or weight-loss program. In addition, some people with type 1 diabetes skip injections to avoid insulin reactions when they are on the starve side of the cycle. That, too, is extremely dangerous.

Bulimia

Another way some people handle a food problem is by becoming bulimic. That means they eat huge amounts

...d they want, then take laxatives or force them-
...omit. They may do this often.

..., which usually occurs in adolescent girls or
...men, is always harmful, and particularly
... for anyone with diabetes. Vomiting and
...ob the body of nutrients. They also violently
...e way you gauge the amount of carbohy-
...ur body has absorbed, leaving no way to
...he amount of insulin needed.

...also causes potassium to be purged from the
...ch may cause severe muscle cramping. Since
...s a muscle, in extreme cases low potassium
...ght on by bulimia can bring on a heart attack.

Anorexia is an eating disorder that also affects mainly
teenage girls and young women. Instead of gorging on
food, then purging, people who are anorexic barely eat
anything at all.

They imagine themselves as being too heavy, even
when they are painfully thin. To lose weight, they barely
eat at all.

Obviously, anorexia is disastrous for healthy diabetes
care.

For More Information

For information about eating disorders, call National Association of
Anorexia Nervosa and Associated Disorders (ANAD) at (847)
831–3438. Or write to them at P.O. Box 7, Highland Park, IL 60035.

ANAD is a non-profit organization established to help and advise people with eating disorders, and their families. It lists the names and
addresses of people who specialize in treating disorders. The list is
arranged by geographical location.

Avoiding an Eating Disorder

An established eating disorder requires professional help by a psychologist, physician, or dietitian to ensure a safe and rapid recovery. As much as family members want to help a loved one return to healthy eating habits, an entrenched eating problem is not something they should try to deal with on their own.

However, there are things that you can do to prevent a food obsession from becoming a food disorder or harming your diabetes control.

* Examine your attitude. How do you feel about your food plan or weight-loss diet? If you feel cheated, deprived, or bitter, take active steps to change your attitude. You might consider seeing a psychologist or other professional.
* Don't install a police officer in your head. Take a flexible attitude toward diet. Rearrange your daily menu whenever possible. Look for variety, interest, and pleasure in the foods you eat regularly. If you do eat something inappropriate, deal with it and move on.
* When food does pop into your mind, make it lead you somewhere else. If the piece of cake you're picturing is going to be served at tonight's party, list three friends who will be there, and something you'd like to say to each. Use the food as an arrow to a "safer topic."
* Set positive, not negative, goals.

Concentrate on what you will do, not what you can't eat.

Non-Food Activities

Any non-food activity will help keep your mind off food. It's difficult to be involved in a physical or mental project while obsessing about foods.

Exercise not only keeps you from thinking about food or consuming it, it also burns calories and strengthens your body. If you exercise enough, you may actually increase your metabolic rate, raising the speed at which you burn calories even when at rest.

If you are a reluctant exerciser, try looking at it as a social activity. Exercise with friends or in a class.

Sports are an even more engaging method of exercise. There are so many organizations sponsoring teams at all levels that it shouldn't be difficult to find something suitable for you—once your doctor gives the OK.

A word of caution: Don't get into something where you sit on the sidelines most of the time. Sports activity, not just interest, is the key.

Helping Others

It's an old axiom that one way to stop thinking about yourself is to help others. There are many people with special needs and all kinds of organizations that are looking for volunteers. Helping someone else may be the best medicine for you.

Contact a religious group, hospital, city or state government, school or university, or ask a librarian where you might volunteer. Young people can volunteer, too, perhaps helping other youngsters learn English, do math, knit, or shoot baskets.

Getting involved in a special interest group, joining a club, or just being with friends can offer absorbing non-food activities.

Although studying hard may seem like too simple an answer, both adults and children have found new priorities for their lives from reading books. Even pets and hobbies can keep your thoughts off food.

The fact is, the busier you are, the less time you have to dwell on what makes you unhappy or bitter, and the less time you have to think about food.

It's clear that there are as many methods of getting rid of the pink polka-dotted elephant as there are people thinking about one. It's not easy, and it takes strong desire on your part. But you can do it.

Cynthia H. Adams, PhD, *is a psychologist and professor of Allied Health Professions at the University of Connecticut in Storrs. She is currently researching eating disorders and diabetes, and has had insulin-dependent diabetes for 10 years.*

7

Yoga for Flexibility & Relaxation

by Nancy Ford-Kohne

It's not a religion. It's not hard. It may be just what you're looking for.

You're stuck in a traffic jam. You've got two options.

Option 1: You begin to feel angry and irritated. You lean on the horn. Within minutes, the famous stress response clicks in. Your heart rate, blood pressure, breathing rate, and blood glucose level goes up. In other words, you and your body are getting ready to "fight or flee." But in a traffic jam, and lots of other situations you face in daily life, you can't fight (who?) or flee (where?).

Option 2: Take a few quieting breaths, put soothing music on the radio or in the tape player. Sit back and do some neck and shoulder rolls if the car is stopped. See the traffic jam as Time Out, a mini-vacation.

Option 2 is yoga in action in your daily life.

Origins in India

Yoga began in India 3,000 to 4,000 years ago. The word "yoga" comes from the Sanskrit language and means, "to join or integrate," or simply "union." Yoga started, as far as we know, as part of India's philosophical system, but not everyone practiced yoga, and it has never been a religion.

About 5 million people in the United States do some yoga. Dance and stretching exercise classes usually have parts and pieces that come directly from yoga. If you ever go to a physical therapist, he or she may give you therapeutic exercises that are yoga postures.

There are several types of yoga. The yoga you may have seen on TV or taught at your local "Y" or an adult education class is called hatha yoga, or physical yoga. Sometimes it's known as the yoga for health. You may also find yoga being taught in a hospital or medical setting. Many health professionals today feel yoga can be part of a treatment plan.

Hatha yoga has three parts: a series of exercises or movements called asana ("poses" or "postures" in English), breathing techniques of all kinds, and relaxation.

Exercises

Yoga exercises strengthen your body and make it more flexible. Yoga also calms your mind and gives you energy. In active sports or strenuous exercises, you use up energy. In yoga classes, students report that they feel tranquil after a class, yet have more energy. Slow and steady motion is the key to going into or coming out of the postures. You hold a yoga pose for several seconds or even minutes and give attention to full, quiet breath. Your yoga instructor will always encourage you to relax as the exercises are being done.

You gently place your body into yoga postures. Done correctly, there's very little chance of injury or muscle stress. A particular asana is not repeated dozens of times, nor are you ever encouraged to push yourself too much.

A yoga session is designed for balance. You stretch to the right and then to the left. You bend back and then forward. You learn to recognize when one side is stronger or more flexible than the other. Thus harmony and balance are achieved with yoga practice.

People of all ages can practice yoga exercises. They are easily modified to meet your needs and physical condition. Don't be put off by the difficult looking postures you may see in a yoga book. A skilled teacher can adapt most asanas by using chairs, cushions, even a wall or other props. A yoga practice can be tailor-made just for you. If something is really impossible for you to do, just forget it. Never compete with yourself or others. Yoga is a stress-free but powerful way to exercise.

Yoga is good for increasing your flexibility and relieving stress, but it doesn't take the place of aerobic exercise. You should still do regular, aerobic exercise, which increases your cardiovascular fitness, helps you lose weight, and, for people with noninsulin-dependent (type 2) diabetes at least, improves blood glucose control.

Breathing and Relaxing

You don't need to fall into the stress mode of life! You can use breath to relax, rather than stress, your mind and body. Yoga helps you to relearn that natural state that your body and mind want to be in: relaxation.

Deep breathing is both calming and energizing. The energy you feel from a few minutes of careful breathing is not nervous or hyper, but that calm, steady energy we all need. Slow, steady, and quiet breathing gives a message to your nervous system: Be calm.

Whole books have been written on yoga breathing. Here is one 5-minute Breath Break. (Read through the instructions several times before you try the practice.)

Hang a "Do Not Disturb" sign on the door. Don't answer the phone. Turn off the radio and TV.

1. Sit with your spine as straight as possible. Use a chair if necessary but don't slump into it. Feet flat on the floor with knees directly over the center of your feet. Use a book or cushion under your feet if they do not rest comfortably on the floor. Hands are on the tops of your legs.

2. Close your eyes gently and let them rest behind closed lids.

3. Think about your ribs, at the front, back, and at the sides of your body. Your lungs are behind those ribs.

4. Feel your lungs filling up, your ribs expanding out and up. Feel your lungs emptying, your ribs coming back down and in. Don't push the breath.

5. The first few times you do this, do it for 2 to 3 minutes, then do it for up to 5 to 10 minutes. At first, set aside a time at least once a day to do this. When you learn how good it makes you feel, you'll want to do it at other times as well.

Just as one stressful situation goes into your next challenge, relaxing for a few minutes every day gradually carries over into the rest of your daily life and activities.

Less Stress

You can look at stress as that little push that gets you moving. Indeed, a little stress that you handle is not the problem—it's when you live with stress every day. The body's response builds up, with no relief. Stress, anxiety, and worry worsen any situation.

When you're stressed, your muscles are tense. A stressed muscle sends more signals of stress throughout the body, making you tense all over. A tense muscle is more prone to injury.

Stress isn't good for your diabetes control either. Stress hormones can raise your blood glucose levels.

Yoga stretches and relaxation techniques are proven ways of coping with stress. While yoga can't make a stressful situation go away, it can change the way you see and respond to that situation. (If you respond with some calmness and tranquillity, the situation itself may become less stressful!)

Gentle yoga stretches help with muscle tension. A muscle can't be stretched and tense at the same time.

Any exercises you now do can be made into yoga exercises: Slow down, hold a position for many seconds, and coordinate your breath and movement. Neck rolls, shoulder rolls, raising and lowering your arms (inhale, arms up; exhale, arms down), and making circles with your ankles and wrists all keep circulation moving. In a beginner yoga class, these kinds of simple exercises are used as warmups.

With slow, progressive movement and stretching, your circulation improves with little or no risk of injury. General cautions with yoga are to stay in your comfort range, don't strain, and never push too hard. Go slowly and steadily, using breathing with the yoga poses or postures. Eventually, with a teacher's help, you can move on to challenging yoga exercises.

While yoga can't make a stressful situation go away, it can change the way you see and respond to that situation.

However, if you have any increased pressure in your eyes (this includes diabetic eye disease and glaucoma), don't do any exercises or poses where your head is lower than your heart. If you have proliferative retinopathy (the more serious form of diabetic eye disease), high blood pressure, or peripheral neuropathy (diabetic nerve disease of the legs and arms), yoga exercises will have to be carefully tailored to your needs. Postures that place your head below your waist will raise blood pressure in your eyes. If you aren't careful to breathe out when you're exerting yourself, your blood pressure will go up. If you have nerve damage, you may overstretch your muscles without realizing it.

Relaxation

Breathing exercises and slow careful stretches are relaxing. In hatha yoga, there is also a separate practice of deep relaxation. Usually at the end of a yoga class, the teacher will lead the class through a progressive relaxation. The teacher will use breathing exercises, guided imagery, and visualization (inhale courage; exhale fear). All these methods help bring about a deep, relaxed state that can carry over into the next several hours.

How to Start

You can get audio or video tapes that give breathing instruction and teach relaxation techniques at health food stores, bookstores, and by mail order. It's probably fine to learn breathing and relaxation from a tape or booklet, but don't try the yoga exercises without a skilled teacher. He or she can make corrections, caution you when necessary, and help you to adapt poses, if you need to.

It will be worth it to you to spend a little time finding an instructor who is right for you. Your diabetes nurse educator or other health care professional may be able to recommend a yoga instructor. Get referrals for a yoga instructor as you would for any professional you might wish to consult.

Yoga instructors aren't required to be certified, but many are, through many different programs. Ask prospective teachers if they are certified. A certified teacher isn't necessarily better than someone who isn't certified, but it's something to consider.

A new organization came into being a few years ago called the International Association of Yoga Therapists. They won't recommend specific instructors but they'll give you a list of institutions, associations, and schools that offer yoga-teacher certification. Through those organizations, you should be able to find certified instructors in your area. For more information, write to the IAYT, Diabetes Committee, at 109 Hillside Ave., Mill Valley, CA 94941 (include a self-addressed, stamped envelope).

Make sure you're working with a yoga teacher who has the training to understand your particular situation. Ask the instructor if he or she has ever worked

Suggested Reading

Gentle Yoga, by Lorna Ben, RN

Easy Does It Yoga For Older People, by Alice Christensen

Yoga for Common Ailments, by Drs. Monro, Nagarantha, and Nagendra with people who have diabetes. If yes, ask the instructor to ask these students to call you. Also, ask if you can observe a class.

If you have any physical problems, you should try a private class where a teacher can design a yoga program for you. Or you should look for a class for seniors, a "gentle" class, or a class in a hospital or physical therapy clinic setting. Private sessions cost about $40 to $60 each; a 10-week group class may cost $50 to $100.

Yoga is fun, healthy, and calming. It's a wise way handed down over several thousands of years. There is little danger in yoga, and even a little progress brings with it freedom and peace of mind.

Nancy Ford-Kohne, MA, *is founder-director of Yoga and Health Studies Center in Alexandria, Virginia. She has been teaching yoga since 1971, and has taught in Europe, Canada, and the former USSR. She is founding president of Unity in Yoga, International, and North American representative for Yoga for Health Foundation, UK. She is certified to teach remedial yoga and is an honorary member of the International Association of Yoga Therapists. She is the American editor for* Yoga for Common Ailments, *published by Simon and Schuster.*

8

Coping With Diabetes

by Irene Pollin

Don't let the
winds of
change
knock you
off your feet.

A year ago you broke your foot and hobbled around in a cast for weeks. A few months ago you had the flu and went to bed for two days, and last week you had a headache, but conquered it in a few hours.

Now you learn you have diabetes and no cast is going to come off and no pills are going to cure you. Your disease is going to be with you the rest of your life, and you are frightened. You may even wonder: Will I be able to do the things I used to do? Will people think differently about me now? Will I get diabetes complications?

You're not alone in those thoughts. Virtually all people who learn they have a chronic illness, no matter their age or sex, walk out of the doctor's office feeling confused and frightened. And, although your doctor has told you it's extremely unlikely complications will occur, you're naturally still pretty nervous about the whole thing.

Rest assured. Your equilibrium will return and you will realize that diabetes can be controlled—once you come to terms with it.

Begin by giving yourself credit for having the brains and ability to make it through life this far. Then realize that those brains and abilities can help you continue to live happily and successfully even with diabetes.

But first, you have to discover your own coping style.

Coping Styles

Although most people have similar fears when they learn they have diabetes, they don't all cope with them the same way. A coping style takes time to develop; you have to work at it. You might even try out a few before you decide which is best for you.

Consider. Would you like to talk about your diabetes to family, friends, and co-workers, or would you rather keep it pretty much to yourself? Would you prefer to plunge into a totally new diet, or choose appropriate foods from those that you are eating now?

Would you like to spend a few weeks being cared for and feeling sorry for yourself, or would you feel more comfortable sitting down and counting your blessings?

Of course, few people remain at one extreme or the other for long. A quiet person may cry openly under certain stresses, and talkers may become alarmingly quiet at times.

Whatever your coping style, it's important to discover it. If you try to fit into someone else's, you'll feel frustrated and ill at ease. You'll also confuse those around you, and rob yourself of a comfortable way of dealing with your world. It's as difficult for the talker to keep his or her feelings quiet as it is for the silent person to talk about them.

Once you find your coping style, accept it. Don't think, "I must be boring everyone pouring out my feelings like this" or "People don't realize I'm hurting inside because I am so quiet about it." In other words, don't fight yourself.

Next, determine the coping style of those around you. That's important, too. If you let your feelings out, but your spouse or children keep theirs in, you may all find yourselves pretty annoyed with each other. Worse, you probably won't realize what is going on. Misunderstanding other people's coping styles can cause tension, arguments, and even breakups between spouses or friends.

If family members don't seem to be reacting to your diabetes as you'd like or expect them to, ask them to sit down and talk about it. You—and they—may be surprised to learn that the difficulties lie not in your feelings, but in your coping styles.

But whatever reaction you get from family members, remember that they are also learning to deal with your diabetes; it affects their lives, too. And don't make the mistake so many people make—deciding that because someone doesn't react to news the way you do that they must not be feeling it as deeply as you.

Integration

The best way to control your diabetes is to integrate it into the rest of your life. No matter how all-encompassing your diabetes regimen may be—and diabetes can be a very intrusive disease—it needn't dominate you unless you let it.

Keeping Your World Turning

Life is going along fairly well. You're making plans, enjoying friends, thinking about the future. Then comes the diagnosis: diabetes.

Suddenly your body requires attention it never required before. Your lifestyle now includes a regimen you don't really want. And you can't envision the future as clearly as you once could.

You may no longer even recognize your own emotions. There's a surge of anger at what has happened, annoyance at having to pay such attention to your health, resentment toward family members who don't have the disease. In short, you feel you've lost control of your life.

While that sense of loss is common among people diagnosed with a chronic illness, each person deals with it in his or her own way.

Some folks immediately make far-reaching decisions such as breaking off an engagement or changing jobs. Others step back, become passive, and let the doctor or a family member tell them what to do. Neither extreme works well in the long run, but here are some methods that do seem to help:

* Separate immediate from long-term problems. Changing the way you eat is an immediate goal. Changing jobs or breaking off a romance is a long-term decision that requires time and perspective to think through.
* Be as involved as possible in your health care. Learn all you can about your type of diabetes. Read books, attend classes, ask questions. Understand why you're supposed to take a certain medication or lose weight or visit an eye or a foot doctor. Participate in your own health care.
* Develop a personal food plan. Work with a registered dietitian, if you can. Walk through a supermarket and read nutrition labels,

study low-fat recipe books, take a cooking class, experiment in the kitchen. Find the foods you like and decide how you will work them into your personal menu.

* Take the lead in helping others adjust to your diabetes. Your family and friends are facing their own anxieties. Step in and explain your disease to them. Let them know you understand their concerns. Ask if they'd like to join you in your new diet or accompany you to an exercise club or on a daily walk.

When you invite them to come to you with their questions abut diabetes, you'll not only appear in control of your life, you'll feel in control, too.

* Maintain a positive self-image. Because part of our self-image comes from the way we perceive our bodies, diabetes can blow a hole in a perfectly solid self-view. Where you once saw yourself as healthy, you may now see yourself as ill. Where you once were independent, you may now need help.

But your new self-image need not be negative. Give yourself credit for tapping strengths you may not have known were there. And make sure the image includes the fact that you are now handling a chronic illness, and you realize that is a courageous thing to do.

* Set goals unrelated to diabetes—then reach them. Have you always wanted to raise roses? Try it. Want to play chess? Find a teacher. Like to take a cruise, dye your hair, grow a beard, make a quilt? Whatever it is, give it a try.

The goal needn't be long term. You'll feel in charge when you set out to wax the car and wind up with a beautifully shiny automobile.

* Plan ahead. Don't drift. Go on with your work, vacations, hobbies, social events. You have a bright and long future. Prepare for it.

The next time you're feeling down, you'll realize that things will get better again.

Yes, diabetes has altered your life. Yes, you have to check your blood glucose, exercise, take medication or insulin, and watch what you eat. And, yes, your diabetes will be there forever.

But so will the rest of your world. Make your disease a part of that world, not its center. Concentrate on activities that have always given you pleasure—films, family, sports, cooking. Keep up with whatever requires your attention—the leaky faucet, an upcoming trip, your homework, a talk in front of your club.

You might actually sit down and list the areas where diabetes conflicts with your previous lifestyle. Does it give you less time to yourself? Does it force you to exercise when you'd rather watch TV? Does it seem to take away all the foods you like?

Then, list possible solutions. You might find some you hadn't thought of before. Perhaps you can set aside an hour during the day or evening when you can put your feet up, read a book, work the crossword puzzle, or do anything you like that is totally unrelated to diabetes.

If you're finding it tough to set aside time to exercise, or if you feel lonely or isolated walking or working out by yourself, invite a friend or family member to get involved, too. Or check out the cost of a health club, or invest in a stationary bike so you can read or watch TV or listen to talking books or music on a headphone while you're sitting in the house cycling.

Look at problems creatively. You might park five blocks away from the house each day, take the stairs, or get off the bus a stop early so you'll get more exercise. You could set up your own food plan that includes some old favorites. You might even eat them during your nondiabetes hour.

The point is, find a lifestyle that keeps you healthy and in charge.

Once you have integrated diabetes into your life, you'll find that it will no longer dominate your world. You'll wake up in the morning and go to sleep at night thinking about the day's activities, not about your disease.

Ebb and Flow

As you adjust to your diabetes over weeks and months and years, remember that adjustment is not like climbing a mountain. You don't go steadily forward until you reach the top. Rather, the process is filled with ups and downs. Some people compare it to riding an ocean wave. Sometimes you are on the crest, sometimes you seem to fall into the trough. Making emotional adjustments requires some flexibility.

Although you can organize the physical steps needed for your diabetes care, you can't determine emotional responses by an act of will. They come in fits and starts. One day you feel upbeat and full of energy and you tell yourself, "I can handle this. Just watch me."

The next morning you wake feeling anxious or depressed, and decide that you'll never be able to keep your diabetes under control.

Or you're sitting alone, thinking that nothing good will ever happen again when the phone rings and someone invites you out. Suddenly, you're feeling fine. That's the nature of emotions. They're constantly changing, especially when you are adjusting to something as new and different as a chronic illness.

Because emotions are so complex and unpredictable, try to face each situation as it occurs. And take comfort in the fact that your emotional swings will become less extreme and less frequent with time.

Time helps in another way, too. Once you have been depressed, then come back up again, you'll begin to recognize the down signs. The next time you're feeling down, you'll realize that things will get brighter again.

One other point. Keep in mind that diabetes isn't the only thing in your life that may be causing you to feel low. After all, you weren't diagnosed in a vacuum. See what else is going on that might be affecting your mood.

Of course, if you have more downs than ups, if your emotions fluctuate wildly, or if you find yourself seriously depressed for days at a time, talk with a mental health or other professional who can offer help.

Remember that you can cope with diabetes. It's not easy, and it's not something you would choose to do—if you had a choice. But, alas, you don't. The wisest move is to face the disease, come to terms with it, then go on enjoying a physically and emotionally satisfying life.

Irene Pollin, MSW, *has specialized in counseling people with long-term diseases and their families since 1974. Pollin has lost two children to chronic illnesses, and is the co-author of* Taking Charge: Overcoming the Challenges of Long-Term Illness.

9
Breaking Free

by Helen Kraus

A positive self-image is the first step toward good health. Learn to accept— even to love— yourself.

Life is tough. Life with diabetes is tougher.

One reason is that our society places a high premium on perfect health. That means that any disease, including diabetes, is quietly frowned upon.

Because of such pressure, some people with diabetes allow their self image to tarnish. Negative thoughts take hold. Unless a person caught up in these feelings recognizes them for what they are—harmful and inaccurate ways of judging him- or herself—the cycle of self-contempt continues.

Have You Noticed These?

Here are a few thoughts that point to low self-esteem. If you catch yourself thinking this way, take note. You may want to take steps to see yourself in a better light.

65

I. Nothing really matters. After all, I have diabetes.
What you're really saying is: My body doesn't work right, so I'm not as valuable as everyone else. If I were really valuable, I wouldn't always have to pay attention to what or when I eat or to how hard I exercise.

Acknowledge
your anger.

The fact is, through no fault of your own, your body has a problem with the way it handles food. That has nothing to do with your value as a human being.

If you look carefully at your friends and neighbors, you'll see that many of them have problems too.

There are those who don't hear well, or who have pains no doctor can diagnose, or who can't retain what they hear or read. Some silently grieve a near-unbearable loss. Others have a dear family member who suffers from an illness that medical science cannot control.

True, some problems are more difficult to bear than others. But we are all human beings, whatever the state of our health, and that alone makes us worthy of respect—especially from ourselves.

2. Why me?
Being diagnosed with diabetes is always a shock. But for some, it's also a message that says, "I must have done something wrong. That's why I'm being singled out for punishment."

That's no surprise.

Again, society plays a part because it values control not only over our bodies, but over our environment and even over the forces of nature. We all strive for such control.

No wonder we think something must be wrong with us when we lose control over something as personal as the way our bodies work.

(You may feel this way even though having your pancreas produce too little or no insulin is clearly not in anyone's control.)

However, if you look deeper at this control question, you'll see something else: anger.

When people lose control over a significant part of their lives, they become angry. In fact, anger is a natural response when you feel that fate or the arbitrary forces of nature have unfairly singled you out.

Unrecognized, buried anger is unhealthy. If you are angry, it's important to be aware of it, to acknowledge it, and to find a positive way to let it out.

Minimizing or covering up anger doesn't rid you of it. It only means you carry it deep inside, where it can eat into you.

Unrecognized anger, for example, can cause you to provoke arguments, and even cause you to harm others or yourself.

One way to diffuse anger is to keep a journal. Then you can spill out your deepest fury while hurting no one. You can also vent your anger in hard exercise or on the playing field. Even joining a debating group or perhaps a political organization—anywhere you can express your feelings—can bring a surprising amount of relief.

3. If I tell people I care that I have diabetes, they won't want to spend time with me. Why would anyone want to get involved with a person who has diabetes?

Movies and TV ads display a parade of young, healthy, beautiful people. And we buy all sorts of equipment and food to make us appear younger and healthier so we can look like this ideal.

But if you have a chronic illness, you are out of synch with the common ideal. No wonder you think people won't like you.

Again, look at the facts. First, you are not unhealthy. You simply have a disease that you must work to control.

Second, you did not bring the disease on yourself, and you are not responsible for having it.

Third, there is no reason to think that having diabetes is something to be ashamed of or to hide.

Yes, diabetes isn't very romantic.

But when you are looking for someone with whom to spend your life, or even someone with whom to spend a significant number of hours, ask yourself: Is this a good relationship if I have to pretend? Don't I want a mate, friend, or lover I can be honest with? Do I want someone who cannot accept me as I am?

Of course, you may not want to tell everyone you meet that you have diabetes right off the bat. And that's fine.

But if you do choose to talk about your diabetes, let people know that you are coping with it well because it is a part of your life, a part of you.

People who care about each other celebrate the whole of the other person. The more aspects of each other you and your friends accept, the greater the likelihood that you will take pleasure in each other and have a close, firm friendship or marriage.

But before you can have such an accepting relationship with someone else, you must first have one with yourself.

4. My blood sugars have shot way up or down (or I can't stay on my food plan). I never do anything right.

Don't sell yourself short by presuming that everything negative relating to your diabetes is caused by you. Yes, this is a self-care disease. But the fact is, neither you—nor your doctor—can completely control it.

Taking care of diabetes is a difficult job; asking for perfection is asking for failure. And failure leads to a poor self-image.

You might do everything that your health care team has spelled out and still have unexplained high or low blood glucose readings.

Although diabetes is a condition that requires taking care of your own health, paradoxically, it also requires acceptance of the fact—again—that some things are out of your control.

Don't deprive yourself of a chance for fun.

So, when your blood glucose numbers don't come out as you think they should, even though you know you have been careful, don't begin to "awfulize." In other words, don't decide that everything is just awful.

When you do that you take a problem and exaggerate it so it becomes all encompassing. That can set a whole cycle of self "put downs" into motion.

When you begin to think you can't do anything right, start listing your positives. Remember the time you handed in a good term paper, prepared a tasty meal, won an award, or even washed the car and made it shine.

Watch out for your own one-sided, negative appraisals. Look for balance in viewing your behavior.

Then take extra credit for the added responsibilities diabetes brings. The world may not know how much work is involved in maintaining good diabetes control, but you do.

5. No one understands.

If you feel that people who don't have diabetes can't possibly understand you, then you are likely to find yourself alone most of the time. After all, that's better than having the rest of the world think something is wrong with you, isn't it?

What's more (you tell yourself) if I tell them about insulin reactions, they'll think I'm real trouble. I better stay away from parties and people who seem to be having a good time.

Whoops. You are not only selling yourself short, but everyone else, too. Don't assume that everyone is locked into such stereotyped thinking. That only deprives you of the chance for fun, and for supportive, nurturing friendships.

Take a chance; open up to others. Sometimes taking a risk enables other people to tell you important aspects of their lives. You may discover that your potential friends have to deal with something out of the ordinary too, and are glad of the chance to talk about it with someone who understands.

Human beings have a wonderful capacity for putting themselves in the other fellow's shoes. Give other people a chance.

It's Up to You

If you are in the dumps about having diabetes, or angry about the unfairness of it all, take steps to deal with these life-draining feelings. You can learn to be at peace with yourself and with this disease.

Always know that you are a valuable, important member of your family, your community, and your world. Diabetes does not measure your value. Your humanity does.

Helen Kraus, PsyD, *is a licensed clinical psychologist in private practice in Cambridge, Massachusetts. She also serves as consulting psychologist at the New England Sinai Hospital and Rehabilitation Center in Stoughton, Massachusetts, and at the Mount Auburn Hospital in Cambridge.*

10
Self-Esteem

by Barbara Cuban

When we think highly of ourselves, others tend to think well of us also.

We've all heard the song, "You're Nobody Til Somebody Loves You," and some of us may actually believe it. But that title says that unless someone else cares about you, you're nothing. The truth is, if you rely on someone else's opinion to define your worth, you're asking for trouble.

We call the definition of our worth our self-esteem, a term hard to define and harder still to measure. You can't touch, smell, see, feel, or taste it. And self-esteem can't be graded with a thermometer or read by a lab test.

So what is self-esteem? It is an internal barometer of the value we place on ourselves. That includes everything from how capable we think we are to our own appearance.

Self-esteem has a strong impact on every part of our lives. We do better in our work, studies, and personal relationships when we have high self-esteem. And we are more likely to go after—and obtain—what we want out of life when we have a strong sense of ourselves and our own worth.

There's a further bonus to evaluating ourselves highly. When we have self-esteem, others are likely to think well of us also.

Beginnings

Although self-esteem has its beginnings early in our lives, we don't seem to be born with it.

Although self-esteem has its beginnings early in our lives, we don't seem to be born with it. We are born with differences in temperament—as infants we respond to our environment in our own way. But our self-esteem appears to form as we bond to parents or caregivers.

Much, although not all, of the way we feel and think about ourselves comes from the way we interpret the messages, spoken and unspoken, that parents and caregivers give us from the time we are very young.

From their treatment of us, we begin to form an opinion of ourselves, an attitude about who we are, and a sense of whether we like or dislike ourselves and in what ways.

For instance, if you were not well coordinated as a child, you might still feel that you are clumsy, unless your parent or caregiver offsets that idea early, perhaps by appreciating other qualities in you.

However, the good news is that psychologists feel that self-esteem is not fixed. In fact, within a certain range, it fluctuates from day to day. We feel better or worse about ourselves depending on things like:

* How we think we look that day
* How others respond to us
* Our physical well-being

* How prepared we are for the day's work
* Whether we feel hopeful or hopeless about the future

Where Does Diabetes Fit In?

Although a high level of self-esteem is difficult for many people to achieve, there can be particular roadblocks to it when you have a chronic disease like diabetes.

For one thing, the physical aspects of diabetes enter the picture. Blood glucose variations can affect your mood, appetite, energy or fatigue level, sense of well-being, and feeling of control over your life.

Some people with diabetes develop low self-esteem because they blame themselves for having the illness. Or, they think less of themselves because they feel different, or wonder if there is something negative that singled them out for this disease.

Be Generous

What can you do to maintain a positive sense of yourself when you have a chronic illness? First, realize that everyone has to deal with some limitations, both actual and believed. Don't be defeated by what you think you don't have or can't do. Focus on your pluses. Be generous with yourself.

The only thing stopping you from having a high self-esteem is your own belief about yourself. Everyone has strengths, so emphasize yours.

When your self-esteem seems low, focus on things you like about yourself—perhaps your participation in a charity drive, the way you patiently explained the homework to a classmate at school, or the fact that you stick to your exercise schedule and food plan. You might also like the way you dress, the handiwork you do, or your ability to enjoy nature. You must refuse to be swallowed up by negative thoughts.

One way to do this is by making a list of things that you like about yourself. If you can't compose such a list, get feedback from others. Keep the list handy for a day when your self-esteem is low.

Negative Myths

Remember, although diabetes can't be eliminated, it can be controlled. And your self-esteem will probably be high when you handle your diabetes well. To do that, it's important to discover any negative myths you may have about yourself.

For instance, you may believe that you can't control your diabetes well because you are a disorganized person who is never prepared for good diabetes self-care.

If you use insulin and don't always carry your monitoring equipment and injection supplies, you feed that image of yourself as disorganized. Then you get upset with yourself, further lowering your self-esteem.

Slowly, you begin to accept the fact that you are disorganized, therefore unprepared and unable to take good care of your health.

However, since everyone has the capacity to be organized and prepared, your view of yourself as a disorganized person is likely to be a myth you have come to believe—a myth that is hurting your self-esteem.

You can disprove such harmful myths in three steps.
* First, recognize them.
* Second, realize that they are myths rather than reality.
* Third, work—with help, if necessary—to change them.

Your self-esteem will probably increase a notch or

two when you discover new abilities you didn't know you have.

The Self-Satisfaction Scale can help you identify areas of low self-esteem. Use it as a guide to help improve your image of yourself.

Also included are tips that can help you raise your self-image. Most of all, remember that self-esteem is learned, therefore it can be changed, and increased.

Self-Satisfaction Scale

Circle the number in each category that best describes yourself. Decide which categories make you feel good about yourself, and which you want to work on.

Category	Low									High
1. Intelligence	1	2	3	4	5	6	7	8	9	10
2. Competence	1	2	3	4	5	6	7	8	9	10
3. Work Performance	1	2	3	4	5	6	7	8	9	10
4. Takes Initiative	1	2	3	4	5	6	7	8	9	10
5. Can Say 'No'	1	2	3	4	5	6	7	8	9	10
6. Accepts Compliments	1	2	3	4	5	6	7	8	9	10
7. Appearance	1	2	3	4	5	6	7	8	9	10
8. Fitness Level	1	2	3	4	5	6	7	8	9	10
9. Ability to Socialize	1	2	3	4	5	6	7	8	9	10
10. Friendships	1	2	3	4	5	6	7	8	9	10
11. Self-Confidence	1	2	3	4	5	6	7	8	9	10
12. Self-Respect	1	2	3	4	5	6	7	8	9	10

How to Improve Your Self-Esteem

Identify what would make you feel better about yourself.

Consider ways you could make those things happen.

Identify something you like about yourself every day.

Associate with people who are supportive and caring about you.

Change your pattern of relating to people who constantly undermine you. Let them know you won't tolerate that negativism anymore.

Tell people directly what you want and what you need, rather than hoping they'll pick up on nonverbal signals.

Give yourself a compliment each day.

Let others know what you like about them. They will start to reciprocate.

Try to have a few enjoyable moments for yourself each day.

If none of these work, consider talking to a professional counselor. Asking for help is a strength, not a weakness.

I Deserve It

You can also raise your self-esteem by acting as if you deserve good health care. When you monitor your blood glucose regularly, take insulin shots on time, do appropriate exercises, and stick with your meal plan—in short, if you act like you value yourself—your self-esteem is likely to go up. That, in turn, will make it more likely that you will continue to take good care of yourself.

Barbara Cuban, LCSW, ACSW, *is a licensed clinical social worker in private practice in Palo Alto, California. Barbara works with individuals, couples, and groups in addition to leading workshops on a variety of subjects such as stress management and self-esteem.*

11

The Problem With Perfection

Healthy
diabetes
control means
practicing the
art of the
possible.

by Susan M. Dallman

"I hate myself when I binge," Julie says. Julie—a teenager with insulin-dependent (type 1) diabetes—is referring to the eating binges she goes on every few months.

Most days Julie stays on her food plan, takes the appropriate insulin dosage, checks her blood glucose, does her exercises, and enjoys fairly good diabetes control.

Then some little thing goes wrong and the binge begins. Julie just can't snap back from even the smallest misstep. "Once I eat even a little more than I should," she explains, "I decide I might as well just go all the way."

Bill is a middle-aged man who has non-insulin-dependent (type 2) diabetes, and is more disciplined than Julie. In fact, he is more disciplined than most people, especially about his diabetes care.

But when Bill tests his blood glucose and finds it higher than he expected—even slightly higher—he feels frustrated and out of control. "What's the use?" he figures, "Nothing I do matters anyway." He winds up ignoring his diabetes regimen, which makes him lose the control he does have.

"What's the use?" Bill figures, "Nothing I do matters anyway."

And then there's Andrea, a young professional woman who has had type 1 diabetes for 15 years. When it comes to sticking with a diabetes program, she has both Julie and Bill beat by a country mile.

Andrea maintains almost perfect blood glucose readings and pays meticulous attention to every facet of her diabetes program. In fact, to make sure all goes well, Andrea doesn't allow herself to eat in restaurants, friends', or even family members' homes; she's afraid any change in her dietary habits will destroy her near perfect control.

The problem is, Andrea has developed a warped social life. She has become isolated from her friends and family who don't understand all the refused invitations.

Why Do We Hurt Ourselves?

None of these people set out to harm themselves, yet they share a self-destructive pattern: their search for perfection. When they bump against the real world where perfection doesn't exist, they feel overwhelmed and out of control. That leaves them with little motivation to manage their diabetes, because they believe managing it is simply impossible.

Of course, everyone with type 1 or type 2 diabetes wants to follow the best regimen. And most do. But the problem with people like Julie, Bill, and Andrea is that they blame themselves for not being perfect.

Julie, for instance, confesses that when she strays from even the smallest element of her diabetes control she feels "bad."

Her binges are not only self-destructive, they reinforce her negative view of herself, and then she punishes herself for being less than perfect.

Bill can't accept the fact that no matter how hard he works, he cannot achieve perfect control. So when things don't go exactly as he thinks they should, he decides that any diabetes care is hopeless and gives up.

While Andrea's self-destructive behavior is more subtle, it also comes from a fear of imperfection. To ward off even the suggestion of failure, she makes her world one dimensional, allowing diabetes to control her life.

This plays havoc with her mental health, breeding isolation and depression. Ultimately, that affects her physical well-being. In addition, she hurts members of her family and friends who would like to be near her.

> Bill can't accept the fact that no matter how hard he works, he cannot achieve perfect control.

Not Unusual

Although Julie, Bill, and Andrea each feels unique, they are actually far from being alone in their self-destructive behavior. The reach for perfection is not uncommon in people with diabetes.

Part of the difficulty lies in the fact that with today's blood glucose self-monitoring, the person with diabetes, not the doctor, is largely responsible for his or her own day-to-day health.

No wonder people become overwhelmed. On top of monitoring their blood glucose, they must also make sure they keep up with their insulin or medication, maintain a food plan or weight-loss diet, and exercise, all while dealing with the everyday stresses of life.

It's no surprise that people who try hard to do the right thing see themselves as failures when one part of the picture doesn't come out just right.

How About You?

Although anyone can have an occasional bout of self-destructive behavior, for some it becomes a pattern that persists for months or years.

Why don't such people ask for help?

Often, they feel guilty or embarrassed. They are afraid people will call them "crazy." Or, they may decide that they really are crazy. After all, as Julie says, "I can't believe I'm doing this to myself, and I'd die if anyone found out."

But when her mother did find out and sought help for her daughter, Julie learned that she was not alone in her negative thoughts about herself. In fact, she discovered that there are a great many other people out there who practice self-destructive behavior to some extent and who think that only crazy people would do such things to themselves.

If you find yourself in an impossible search for perfection, or a cycle of self-destructive behavior, here are some steps that may help you break the pattern.

Ask for help. You may need more support than friends or family can provide. The least expensive kind of help is likely to come from a diabetes support group. Such groups may be free or very inexpensive. See chapters 17 and 25.

You may be able to locate one through your local ADA Affiliate, religious leader, physician, Certified Diabetes Educator, Registered Dietitian, or a friend.

If you want more private or more professional attention, ask the same sources for a therapist who specializes in issues related to chronic illnesses.

It's important that the therapist—whether he or she is a social worker licensed by a state board of mental health (LCSW) or accredited by the national Academy of Certified Social Workers (ACSW), a psychologist (PhD), or a psychiatrist (MD)—has training in the area of self-destructive behavior and chronic illnesses. Together, you can work on discovering the underlying issues that may be preventing you from managing your diabetes while maintaining good mental health.

Some insurance plans may cover this therapy as part of your diabetes care, rather than under a separate "mental health benefits" category.

Try for more flexibility. The more choices and flexibility you have, the more in control you will feel.

Doctors find that people who don't feel deprived of foods they enjoy are most likely to stick with a food plan or weight-loss diet. Julie, for instance, felt that she was never permitted to stray from her food plan. It followed that she had to be "bad" to eat something not on the list. Once she became "bad," she couldn't shake the negative image of herself.

You can avoid such self-destructive behavior by talking with your doctor and registered dietitian about introducing some flexibility in your diabetes regimen, such as increasing your food choices or scheduling an occasional high-calorie snack, even if you are on a weight-loss diet.

Scheduling the snack or extra food also allows you and your doctor to work out an appropriate insulin dosage to cover the occasional change.

Be open. Your emotions, struggles, depressions, and even self-destructive behavior should not be a cause of shame or embarrassment. You are better off listening to what your behavior is telling you, not hiding from or ignoring the message. Your feelings will not go away if you ignore them.

However, it's good to know that you have a lot more company than you might expect and a lot more compassion and understanding available than you might realize.

Be realistic. Establish realistic goals. Don't expect perfect blood glucose readings every hour of every day. That's just not going to happen to human beings. Neither will you be able to eat the same food at precisely the same time or maintain the same level of activity every day. Those are not realistic goals and expecting to achieve them will only lead to unhappiness.

There are limits as to how much control anyone can have over diabetes, or any other aspect of their health, for that matter.

Don't misuse your diabetes tools. Remember, blood glucose readings are your tool, not your master. They were developed to free you from some of the limitations of diabetes, not to make you strive for the impossible. If you think of imperfect blood glucose readings as cause for punishment, you are letting the tail wag the dog.

Sometimes, despite your best efforts, you just won't get the readings you want, because there are many factors that influence blood glucose levels, and a good many of them are simply out of your control.

Don't make your diabetes regimen become a cause for self-blame, isolation, or depression. Take a look at how you are handling your diabetes treatment, and make good mental health as much of a goal as good physical health.

Susan M. Dallman, LCSW, ACSW, *is currently working with The Family Advocacy Program at Lowry Air Force Base in Denver, Colorado.*

12
Getting the Best of Stress

Do you think stress is a fact of life? There's plenty you can do to change that "fact."

by Barbara Cuban

Stress—psychological, emotional strain, tension—seems so common today it's been called the disease of the 90s. Many of us feel we have no choice but to feel stressed by the world we live in.

The good news is that much of the stress we feel is not something done to us from "out there;" it's a feeling we create within ourselves. Stress is our own internal response to the situation of the moment, as well as to messages recorded within us a long time ago. Because much of stress comes from within, we can often control it. But it takes work.

Certainly there are external pressures—deadlines, ringing telephones, traffic tie-ups that make our stomachs churn. The only people who aren't affected by these pressures are in cemeteries.

Stress, in fact, is part of life. Remember the flight-or-fight response? That's when adrenaline flows faster and allows us to move quickly. The pupils dilate, the heart beats faster, the palms sweat. Once, this response probably allowed us to escape from wild animals or other dangers. We still need that fast flow of adrenaline when we dart across a street avoiding traffic, or when we have a special job to get done quickly. But we don't need it all the time.

Personality Types

In learning to handle stress, the first thing to realize is that not everyone finds the same things stressful, and not everyone responds to stress the same way.

You've probably heard about type A and type B behavior personalities. These personality types are one way to contrast varying responses to situations, to other people, even to our own thoughts.

Type A folks are usually in a hurry. They're impatient with themselves and others and tend to overschedule and do more than one thing at a time. Type As are often competitive and are likely to be perfectionists. They are generally hostile men and women who hold onto their anger.

On the other hand, type B personalities rarely feel the urgency of time. They pace themselves, don't overreact, and can say "no" if they're too busy to take on a new assignment. They're usually modest about their achievements and don't need to produce to feel good about themselves.

Of course, most of us have some type A as well as type B characteristics. But these personality types make it easy to see that stress is created by the way we react to a situation, not by the situation itself.

Stress and Diabetes

Scientists tell us that stress may be a factor in heart disease and stroke. Because diabetes is also a risk factor in these diseases, it's particularly important for people with diabetes to learn ways to handle their stress.

In addition, diabetes can magnify stress. In fact, diabetes carries its own stressors. Being diagnosed with either insulin-dependent (type 1) or non-insulin-dependent (type 2) diabetes can churn up real, imagined, or expected stresses. It can make you feel your body is no longer under your control. It may lower your self-esteem (something is wrong with me) or cause anger (why me?), guilt (I must have done something wrong), depression (I feel sad and hopeless), or helplessness (I can't cope with this). Such stressful thoughts can have a powerful effect on the body.

Diabetes can bring on stressful external situations, too. These might include the way friends, family, or co-workers perceive you and your disease; the cost of medical care; strict dietary limitations; and the need to carry supplies everywhere. If you take insulin, you may find injections stressful. If you are non-insulin-dependent, needing to lose weight and exercise may be hard to deal with.

Although maintaining control over the disease is important for people with diabetes, trying too hard also isn't a good idea. It can lead to disillusionment—more stress. If you are a type A personality and expect to deal absolutely perfectly with diabetes, you're setting yourself up for a high-anxiety scenario.

Choices

Although many people with diabetes may have similar feelings, they choose different ways of responding to them.

Denying that diabetes is a serious disease is one choice some people make. So is keeping haphazard control of diabetes.

Sometimes people choose to fight stress through ways that actually worsen the problem. They may turn to alcohol, prescription medications, illegal drugs, caffeine, nicotine, or anything that will either give them a lift or calm them.

Some choose food binging as a way to fill the empty space inside. In fact, any excessive behavior, even gambling or oversleeping, may be a way to deal with stress.

Although few of these solutions work long for anyone, when you have diabetes most of them are dangerous from the word "go." They alter diabetes control and endanger health. But learning as much as possible about diabetes, becoming an expert in your body's responses, and cooperating with your health care professionals are choices some people make.

When you have diabetes, it pays to look hard for healthy ways to deal with feelings of loneliness, low self-esteem, anger, other uncomfortable emotions, or outside pressures.

Managing Stress

Everyone has stress. There are, however, ways to feel less stressed and ways to manage the stress you do feel.

Some symptoms of stress include:
* frequent and prolonged boredom
* prolonged frustration

Progressive Relaxation

The purpose of this technique is to achieve complete relaxation all through the body by relaxing groups of muscles in sequence. Start with the facial muscles, then work down to your feet and toes. As you identify each group of muscles, tense them. Coordinate the tension with your breathing. Keep your eyes closed and imagine yourself relaxing.

1. Close your eyes and breathe slowly and deeply.

2. Inhale. Raise eyebrows. Tense them. Hold for the count of three. Relax eyebrows. Exhale.

3. Inhale. Close mouth and eyes tightly. Squeeze. Hold for the count of three. Relax eyes and mouth. Exhale.

4. Inhale. Bite down on teeth. Hold for count of three. Relax jaw. Exhale.

5. Inhale. Pull shoulders up. Hold for count of three. Relax shoulders. Exhale.

6. Inhale. Tense all muscles in the arms. Hold for count of three. Relax arms. Exhale.

7. Inhale. Tense all muscles in the chest and abdomen. Hold for count of three. Relax muscles. Exhale.

8. Inhale. Tense all muscles in the legs. Hold for count of three. Relax muscles. Exhale.

9. Inhale. Tense all muscles in toes. Curl toes. Hold for count of three. Relax the muscles. Exhale.

10. Keep your eyes closed for a short while. Gradually open them.

* crying spells
* frequent self-criticism
* nervous laughter
* easy discouragement
* emptiness
* apathy

First, find out what causes your body to feel stressed. Diabetes testing can help you there. Test your blood glucose levels when you are in—have just come out of—a stressful situation. That will tell you how the event affected your blood glucose levels, which will help you see what situations are stressful for you.

More insight might come from deciding whether you are more of a type A, or type B personality. If you're type A, make a contract with yourself to slow down and to stop overcommitting your time. Get oth-

Meditation

This technique is good when you are feeling rushed and need to slow yourself down.

1. Choose a quiet environment where you will not be disturbed.

2. Get into a comfortable position.

3. Close your eyes.

4. Deeply relax your muscles.

5. Breathe through your nose. As you breathe out, say the word "one" to yourself.

6. Keep repeating this for 10 to 20 minutes.

7. When you have finished, allow yourself to sit quietly for a few minutes longer before opening your eyes.

ers to help out, and learn to say "no" when you feel like it. Allow extra hours to get things done and block out some time just for yourself.

Exercise is a natural anti-stress aid. Before you start a regular exercise regimen, ask your doctor how it might change your insulin or diet needs. It's good to vary your exercises so you don't get bored, and always start by warming up, then slowing down gradually. Then slowly increase your endurance and stamina.

Here are some other ways to help handle stress:

* Find someone to talk to when something is bothering you.
* Join a support group.
* Form a discussion group on books, movies, or whatever interests you.
* Join a bowling league or get into some sport activity.
* Start a potluck dinner group.
* Join a dance group—square dancing, jazz, folk, tap, ballroom.
* Take up a hobby like stamp or coin collecting or needlepoint.
* Sign up for a class.
* Learn to play a musical instrument.
* Volunteer to help others.
* Take mini-vacations, overnighters, or weekends away.
* Arrange for baby-sitters when you're home to allow for free time.
* Form a baby-sitting cooperative with other parents so you can get out more.

Everyone has choices in life. Pace yourself. Avoid excessive behavior. Make it a point to identify your stressors and do something about them. You may not be able to control traffic jams, an angry boss, or a crying baby, but you do have some control over your reactions to them. You even have control over how you react to your diabetes.

Barbara Cuban, LCSW, ACSW, *is a licensed clinical social worker in Palo Alto, California, where she has a private practice. She works with individuals, couples, and groups in addition to leading workshops on a variety of subjects such as stress management.*

13
The Last Laugh

by Wendy Satin Rappaport

Ever stub your toe on the same chair three times in a row, then burst out laughing? Or grabbed your lunchbag as you raced out of the house, discovered you'd snatched the onions, and guffawed at your mistake?

Your humor may have done more than save a bad moment. It might have helped your body fight an old and dangerous enemy—stress. For people with diabetes, that's no laughing matter.

When you have diabetes, stress can send blood sugar levels soaring or cause you to ignore your diabetes regimen. And stress is a recognized factor in heart disease and stroke, an especially important fact to people with diabetes, who have above-average vulnerability to those diseases.

Humor can buffer against stress. When we can't control an event, humor can still let us control the way we view it.

Long Laugh Line

"Men are disturbed not by things but by the view which they take of them."

Epictetus

The notion that humor is good therapy for some diseases and for what we call stress has a long, respected history. Even in ancient times, physicians noted that humor helped their patients improve.

More recently, Norman Cousins, Editor Emeritus of Saturday Review and Adjunct Professor of UCLA School of Medicine, took a heavy dose of humor to help himself fight symptoms of a serious illness, ankylosing spondylitis. Cousins checked into a hotel and regularly viewed comedy films as he lay ill. He found that 10 minutes of laughter gave him several hours of pain-free sleep without medication.

Although there might have been biological causes for Cousins' improvement, he isn't alone in believing humor played a part.

It's not hard to see why humor should help the body fight some diseases and stress. Humor has been called a kind of "internal jogging" that helps the mind relax by relieving a sense of frustration or disappointment. And it does this in a socially acceptable manner.

It's also not hard to see why humor might be an especially effective ally in handling a chronic disease like diabetes.

For one thing, there is an emotional element in diabetes. The diagnosis itself, daily management of the disease, feelings of vulnerability, and fears of the future it often brings can create resentment, anger, and anxiety. Those feelings may, in turn, affect diabetes control.

Scientists are quick to caution us, however, that

humor's effect on the body is difficult to calculate, and that it's different in different people.

You may have seen people with diabetes who seem to have no obvious significant emotional problems, yet remain in poor control of their disease. Then there are others who seem to have a great deal of stress, but seem to stay in good control.

Apparently certain people are able to defend themselves from the effects of stress. Scientists believe something in their individual personalities—a kind of mental hardiness—protects them.

For the rest of us, stress seems to play some part in how our bodies react to illness. Poorly handled stress may reduce the immune system's ability to fight disease, but relaxation may help it. In areas like these, stress-reducing humor could play an important role.

Charting the Chuckles

There are varying theories of how humor works. Freud thought that when a difficult emotion is given an outlet, it reduces tension. He called humor, "a pleasurable discharge of a painful effect," a kind of "necessary and healthy internal debunking process."

Other psychiatrists consider humor more mental, less emotional. According to this view, laughter works its magic by helping us link two ideas or events that have nothing in common, letting us see things in a new and lighter way: "I call that dress my diabetes diet diving suit. Whenever I wear it, I remember not to go off the deep end."

Humor can also provide a new perspective on a negative situation. That external perspective helps us stay outside the situation, rather than being in the middle of it, which helps reduce anxiety or anger.

Humor, used well, is a valuable tool to help master the parts of our lives that seem beyond our control.

Humor can let us show superiority, helping us combat the feelings of inferiority and vulnerability that a chronic illness often brings: "Whenever I see the boss get here, I take my insulin shot because I know it's lunchtime."

Or you might feel amused when you give yourself a shot in a public bathroom and you know people are thinking, "What a nice person to be on drugs."

With humor we can spout our feelings of anger or annoyance without expressly stating that we're angry or annoyed. That allows us to release stress in an acceptable way: "Can you eat that?" someone might ask.

"Why? Is the cook that bad?"

Humor also smoothes the social scene. When you have diabetes, it can help you deal openly with personal interactions you might not be able to handle more directly. If you're working or going to school, maintaining good diabetes control can be related in part to having good social skills. They can help you follow your diabetes regimen wherever you are, and whoever you are with, while keeping your stress level down.

For instance, when you have diabetes you might feel there is a barrier between yourself and others. That can make it difficult to have lunch with classmates or the office gang. You might stay away from social functions or even a company picnic because of that feeling.

The difficulty could relate to the fact that you don't just choose your food casually like the rest of the crowd. Perhaps you fear displaying some unusual behavior. Or maybe you're defensive about peer pressure to eat or drink more. It could also be your concern about taking shots or monitoring blood sugar in front of friends or having low blood-sugar symptoms like irritability or sweating.

But humor can break such barriers because humor brings openness. It also tells people you aren't overly conscious about your diabetes, that it's not something they should be nervous about, that it doesn't make you unapproachable: "Why don't you sit at my table at the banquet? If the service is slow, I can always tell them I need to be served right away because I have diabetes."

Then there is the humor that helps buffer against something frightening. Woody Allen uses this kind to work out fears and to accept the unchangeable. Here's how he handled a subject that's rough for everybody. "I'm not afraid of death. I just don't want to be there when it happens."

Humor can help us respond to thoughtless diabetes-related questions: "What are you doing with that slice of cake? You have diabetes, don't you?"

"Oh, is that what it is? I thought it was a paper-weight." Or perhaps you think, but don't say, "You look as if you've been eating a lot of it."

A light response can lower the anger level and bring some release from the feeling of being patronized.

The Flip Side

Humor, however, like so many factors that affect the mind, can be a two-way street. The downside is that humor can be a defense against reality. It can let someone deny the importance of an illness, and so refuse to get help for it. It can help avoid things we don't want to face, like the fact of a chronic disease or the need to watch our diet.

Humor, used well, is a valuable tool to help master the parts of our lives that seem beyond our control.

But, you say, I'm just not funny, and I never was the life of the party? Not to worry. The good news is that it is possible to get better at using humor in a positive way by practicing it. You don't have to have an innate ability to make people laugh to look for the odd side of a situation.

You can also take your humor from outside sources. See a funny movie, read a joke book, or watch a comedian on television. Keep on the lookout for the offbeat side of events.

Being funny is not as necessary as thinking funny.

And the next time things get a little tense, turn to your neighbor and say, "Now take my diabetes—please."

Wendy Satin Rappaport, PhD, ACSW, *is Assistant Professor of Medicine at the Diabetes Research Institute, University of Miami Medical School.*

14

What's Your Coping Style?

How to use
your natural
style of coping
when control
gets difficult

by Lee S. Schwartz

If you have diabetes, you can probably remember a time—perhaps many times—when your blood-sugar levels have gone out of control for no apparent reason. Ups and downs in control can make you feel like you're on an emotional roller coaster.

Some people seem to have a knack for weathering the frustrations that these episodes of poor control bring on. They keep their calm while they work with their health care team to restore balance.

Fortunately, there's no magic in how these people stay so levelheaded. Their secret is that they know how they cope best and know how to use that coping style to their advantage.

Periods of inexplicable poor control bring out different responses in different people. One way to look at how loss of control affects you is by assessing your coping style. Complete the quiz on page 101 to find out whether your coping style is inner directed or outer directed.

Inner-directed people tend to see themselves as responsible for everything that happens to them. Feeling in control of things that happen around them is very important. When it comes to diabetes, inner-directed people like to feel that they are in control of their blood sugar levels.

When inner-directed people suddenly confront an inexplicable episode of poor control, they spring into action. They try even harder to assert control. They work to make things right by testing more often, eating less (or more), exercising less (or more), or changing insulin dosage. As all attempts to bring the diabetes under control prove fruitless, frustration mounts. But still, the inner-directed person cannot give up the need to control a situation that is, at least temporarily, beyond control. As their anger over the situation builds, they focus their rage inward, blaming themselves for circumstances out of their control. The result is often depression, feelings of powerlessness, and even more frustration.

Outer-directed people, on the other hand, tend to see other people as responsible for what happens to them in life. An abrupt loss of control will send outer-directed people to their doctor for direction. Rather than trying to take control themselves, outer-directed people will become more dependent on the doctor. During bouts of poor control, they may visit the doctor more and more often. They'll put increasing pressure on the doctor to solve what appears to be—at least for the time being—an unsolved riddle.

When nothing seems to work, both the person with diabetes and the doctor become increasingly frustrated. The doctor may start to feel burdened by the numerous calls asking for answers that—for the moment—are unobtainable. Dissatisfied with the doctor's advice, the person with diabetes may seek advice elsewhere. When others, too, are unable to help, anger and frustration increase. Outer-directed people may transfer their angry feelings to their doctor or family members, blaming them for not making things right. In turn, the physician or family member may react with annoyance. The outer-directed person, who looks to others so much, then begins to feel depressed and helpless, as those important others withdraw.

Which Are You?

Perhaps you recognize parts of yourself in the inner-directed person and the outer-directed person. Few people are either completely one or the other. At different times and under different circumstances, you may respond one way or another. During a bout of poor control, you may find you sometimes behave like an inner-directed person and sometimes like an outer-directed one. It may help you to have a sense of the mode in which you're responding. Once you do, you'll be able to put that knowledge to work for you.

If, in general, you see yourself as inner directed—a person who needs to feel in control—your main task is to increase your sense of control in areas of your life over which you continue to have power. Here are some suggestions for when your diabetes goes out of control:

* Try to divert attention away from the diabetes onto things that can be controlled. For example, you may be in the middle of a project at work or at home.

Wrapping up that assignment or finishing building those shelves can give you a sense of mastery and completion in one area of your life.

* Plan and do things that you enjoy and that make you happy. Buy tickets for a play or movie, treat yourself to a new book or record, or buy yourself flowers or a new plant for your house.

* Redirect your thinking about blood sugar tests. For the time being, stop worrying about achieving perfect control. Instead, just take things day by day. Use each blood sugar test as a way to normalize your blood sugar at the moment. By responding to each test, you'll be reasserting your sense of mastery and control.

If, on the other hand, you see yourself as an outer-directed person—someone who wants to be directed—your goal should be to expand your helpful contacts with other people. You may find the following suggestions helpful:

* Arrange short but regular phone or office consultations with your doctor. This way you won't feel like a bother, and your doctor can plan for more frequent contact.

* Give family and friends specific suggestions for helping you. Remember to spread out your requests for support, so that you're not overwhelming one family member.

* Ask people in your diabetes support group for help. Others who've been through the same frustrations can often offer the best support.

* Make social contacts that can help keep your morale up and help you relax. Plan activities or outings with friends.

Keep in mind that occasional times of disturbed control, when nothing seems to have changed and nothing seems to help, are part of having diabetes and being on

How Do You Cope?

At times, we all face situations over which we have no apparent control. These situations offer a chance to assess your coping style. Do you tend to react as an inner-directed or outer-directed person? Complete the following quiz and see.

1. You've studied all semester and feel well-prepared for your final exam. When you receive a failing grade you:
   A. Blame yourself and try to figure out what you did wrong.
   B. Blame your study group and teacher for not reviewing very thoroughly.

2. You are passed over for a well deserved promotion. You:
   A. Take yourself to task and resolve to set higher standards for yourself and work even harder.
   B. Try to find out what is going on in the company that you don't know about.

3. When you miss a deadline for a big project at work, you:
   A. Feel frustrated with your department and wish that your boss hadn't been out when you needed her input.
   B. Feel upset with yourself and review your planning schedule, looking for ways you could have miscalculated.

4. You splurge on an expensive outfit, but when you get home you discover it doesn't fit properly. You:
   A. Are disgusted with yourself. Why didn't you notice the problem when you tried on the outfit?
   B. Are annoyed at the salesperson. After all, you asked specifically if the outfit looked all right.

5. You're denied credit from your bank. You call the bank manager to ask:
   A. How they could have misread your application.
   B. If you did anything wrong filling out the application.

6. You've planned a big family reunion at a local picnic area. Everyone's having a good time when a sudden storm breaks out. Only then do you discover that there's no shelter in the area. You:
   A. Think the park is poorly planned. How could they forget to include a shelter?
   B. Feel embarrassed. Why didn't you think to check about shelter ahead of time?

7. You've just gotten a haircut that you absolutely hate. You think:
   A. Why didn't I bring a picture or explain more clearly what I wanted.
   B. Look what they did to me!

8. You are late for work and can't find your house keys. You:
   A. Blame yourself for not putting them in the usual spot.
   B. Wonder who moved your keys.

9. You've just finished painting your living room and to your dismay the color isn't want you wanted. You:
   A. Knew you should have painted a test patch to make sure the color was right.
   B. Knew you should never have relied on that salesman in the paint store.

10. You're late for an appointment. You start your car and notice that the gas gauge is on empty. Now you'll have to stop for gas. You:
    A. Are angry at your family. Who used the car last and forgot to fill up the tank?
    B. Are upset with yourself for not planning better and allowing more time to make it to your meeting.

Scoring: For questions 1, 2, 4, 7, 8, and 9, give yourself 1 point for every B and no points for every A answer. For questions 3, 5, 6, and 10, give yourself 1 point for every A and no points for every B answer. The higher your score, the more outer directed your coping style. The lower your score, the more inner directed your style.

insulin. Medical science says that control is something that the person with diabetes should aim to achieve to the highest degree.

But tight control all of the time is not realistic. While insulin-dependent diabetes can usually be well-controlled, ups and downs do occur. These are trying times, but they are also times you can find the strength to tolerate and surpass.

***

Lee S. Schwartz, MD, *a clinical associate professor of psychiatry and behavioral sciences at Northwestern University Medical School, is in private practice in Chicago.*

15
Anger

by Lorraine L. Cook

How to make this misunderstood emotion work for you.

We've all felt it—heart-pounding, temple-throbbing, fist-clenching anger. The words we use to describe anger show how we view it. We get steamed, blow our stack, fly off the handle, have a conniption. We think of angry people as out of control, belligerent, irrational. Anger is the black sheep of emotions. But the fact is, anger can be necessary and beneficial. The capacity to become angry is an impressive gift that is part of our biological inheritance. Anger helps us assert and protect ourselves. Without anger, we would be helpless in the face of countless difficulties.

Though anger can be an uncontrolled, destructive force, it also helps preserve and enhance our lives. We can learn to put the power of our anger to constructive use.

What Is Anger?

Anger is a physical state of readiness. Because we are trained to listen to our bodies, those of us with diabetes are usually well-attuned to what happens physiologically when we're angry. More adrenaline is secreted, more sugar is released, our heart beats faster, our blood pressure rises, the pupils of our eyes dilate, and we are highly alert. When we are angry, our bodies are well primed for action.

Why do we get angry? The answer seems simple: We get angry because someone (or thing) makes us mad. But there's more to it than that. When anger occurs, two things are present: a person and a threat. When we feel anger, we feel—in some way—threatened or in danger.

Generally speaking, we get angry when we see an event or person as a threat to our basic survival needs (food, water, shelter) or our more advanced psychological needs (identity, adequacy, recognition, achievement, respect, social affiliation).

Diabetes, whether it's type 1 or type 2, is the perfect breeding ground for anger. First there is coping with the initial diagnosis. "Why me?" many people ask. "It's so unfair!"

Take, for example, Mary H. Her feelings six months after diagnosis are not unusual. "I am angry! I don't want this disease. I don't want to treat it. I don't want to control it. I hate it!"

Diabetes can make us feel threatened. The diagnosis can bring fear of insulin reactions, hyperglycemia, and future complications. Living with diabetes means lifestyle changes—giving up foods we love, following a treatment schedule, monitoring blood sugar levels—that can threaten our self-esteem.

For Mary H., an attractive woman in her mid-fifties, the diagnosis represented not only a threat to her life, but to her lifestyle and self-esteem. A very proud woman, active in community and social affairs, she found it impossible to admit her "weakness." She did not want her hostesses to have to prepare special plates or desserts for her. Denial was her chief defense, and, of course, her blood sugar control was poor. She even felt her husband regarded her as an "invalid" and that she was "less of a woman" in his eyes. In Mary's case, denial fueled her anger at the disease.

For Mary, as for many of us, anger is our main defense when we feel threatened. Instead of putting her anger to work for her, Mary remained locked in what Hendrie Weisinger, PhD, calls the anger circle.

Caught in the Circle

Typically, people respond to a threat or danger with an "anger circle" of thoughts, bodily changes, and behavior. Here's how it happens. You are driving in rush hour traffic and a car suddenly changes lanes, cutting you off. You feel threatened and react with angry thoughts. "What is that idiot doing?" you think. Your body reacts to these thoughts with pounding heart and tensed muscles. You interpret these body signals of anger arousal as further evidence of anger, thinking, "This infuriates me! He almost hit me." The next thing you know you are pounding on the horn and yelling out the window.

When you realize how tense and upset you feel, you may become even angrier. "He made me so angry," you think, blaming the other driver. In fact, you make yourself angry. Observing your "self" doing these angry actions further fuels your anger and intensifies each reaction. Our own thoughts, bodily changes, and behavior build our anger—not someone else's action or an external event.

Saying "You make me angry" is self-defeating. You are abdicating control and giving someone else power over you. In blaming your anger on someone else or on a daily event, you give up the chance to change how you respond.

Breaking the Anger Circle

Rather than staying stuck in the anger circle, you can learn to read your anger signals and use the power of your anger to break the circle.

This three-part approach, suggested in Dr. Weisinger's *Anger Work Out Book*, often helps:

* Identify what is triggering your anger and understand how anger affects your life.
* Change the thoughts, physical responses, and actions that fuel your anger.
* Substitute productive ways to deal with your anger.

Easier said than done? Let's consider an approach that might help Mary H. To understand her anger and make it work for her, she first needs to identify what triggers her anger. One way to do this is with an anger diary, as Neil Clark Warren suggests in his book, *Make Anger Your Ally*. Mary began to keep a record of her angry feelings. Each evening, she sat down and thought about the times she'd felt angry during the day. She started every diary entry with the date and time. Then she noted the following: Who was I angry with? Why was I angry? How did I react?

By keeping the diary, Mary found that she often became angry at social gatherings when friends made a point of asking her what she could eat or hostesses made special foods for her. She was angry because she did not want to be treated differently in public. Usually, she reacted by becoming uncharacteristically silent and withdrawn. Soon she began turning down invitations. As a result, she started to feel "cut off" from her friends.

Reading her diary entries, Mary also noticed that she became angry with her husband when he mentioned her diabetes. When she asked herself why she felt angry, she discovered it was because he seemed to always think of her in terms of her disease. She began to see a pattern to their arguments. They usually occurred at mealtimes and went like this:

TOM: The Jeffersons invited us to dinner on Saturday. I told Arthur it sounded fine.

MARY: I wish you'd checked with me first.

TOM: Check? What's to check? They're our oldest friends, and we haven't seen them for weeks.

MARY: I'd just like to be consulted first.

TOM: Don't you want to go?

MARY: Not particularly.

TOM: Why not?

MARY: I just don't. I won't be able to eat anything anyway...

TOM: I'm sure Betty would fix something for you...

MARY: No! That's exactly the problem. I don't want her to. It's too complicated.

TOM: I don't think Betty would mind. Why she even asked what you could have...

MARY: Oh, this is great. You and Betty talking about my diabetes. What else did you discuss? My latest blood-testing results? My weight? I wish everyone would just leave my diabetes out of it.

TOM: Look, Mary, I just thought you'd enjoy an evening out, but if you don't feel up to it...

MARY (stiffly): I'd rather stay home. You go if you want.

TOM: Forget it. We'll stay home.

These arguments leave Mary feeling both angry and guilty. She's angry because she feels that Tom and her friends now just think of her in terms of her diabetes. She's also afraid that Tom will resent her for not wanting to go out. She's guilty because she's certain that Tom blames her diabetes for imposing changes on their lifestyle.

By identifying the situations in which she became angry, Mary began to see how anger was controlling her life. In social gatherings, which she had always enjoyed, anger made her unhappy and sullen. It was also driving a wedge into her marriage. And its effects on her blood sugar levels were showing up in erratic self-testing results. Mary decided that it was time to break the anger circle. Her first step was to change her physical reaction to events that produced anger. In social situations, she knew that her whole body felt tense as she became angry. She could feel her face become hot and flushed. At home, she often started to speak louder and more quickly with her fists clenched.

Mary found a way to call "time out" for herself when she felt these early warning signs of anger. Her plan was simple: she'd count to 20 every time she felt herself becoming angry and concentrate on slow, steady, deep breathing. She was giving herself time to think and not just react.

Like Mary, many people with diabetes have an unusual ability to sense physical changes and change their responses. Perhaps that's because they are used to monitoring blood sugars and usually know when they are stressed. They know that when their body talks, they need to listen and respond. But when caught up in anger arousal, they may forget to listen.

Here are some ways to calm yourself when you feel anger arousal taking over:

* Talk more slowly. Did you ever hear anyone yell slowly?
* Breath longer and more deeply. This helps calm you.
* Get yourself a drink of water. This will literally help you cool off.
* If you are standing, sit down. Sitting down helps quash your anger arousal and makes you more comfortable.
* If you are sitting down, lean back. When you're yelling, leaning forward is part of the fighting posture.
* Keep your hands at your sides. Shaking your fists and waving your arms speeds up your circulation.
* Quiet yourself. Silence is golden in these situations.

Mary came to understand that changing your thoughts doesn't mean that you stop feeling angry. Rather, you concentrate on not letting your angry thoughts spiral out of control. Changing your physical responses and actions can help. (Try the "Breaking The Circle" exercise below.)

As you break the anger circle, you'll want to channel your angry feelings into more productive uses. Mary did this by adding new entries to her anger journal. Every time she felt angry, she asked herself: What did I want to accomplish with my anger? How did I act on my plan?

Mary decided that when the subject of her diabetes came up in social situations, she would answer the questions in a matter of fact way to try to educate her friends about the disease. (Many of them thought that diabetes meant avoiding carbohydrates and eating a special bland diet.) However, after several attempts, she found that she could not make her plan work; having her diabetes discussed in public made her furious.

At that point, Mary realized that she had still not accepted that fact of having diabetes. To get more support, she joined her local ADA chapter. Meeting other people with diabetes helped her realize that having dia-

Breaking the Circle

1. List the last two times you were angry. What made you angry?

2. How did you feel? Afraid, threatened, hurt, or frustrated?

3. What did you think and say when you got angry?

4. Go back to your list of what you did and said when you were angry. Check the anger actions.

5. List the bodily changes that you are aware of when angry. Begin to use them as a cue to take a deep breath, count to 10, or whatever else helps you "buy time."

6. The last time you were angry, what did you want to accomplish? List two things you could have done to help you accomplish your goal.

7. The next time you are angry, ask yourself, "How can I make my anger constructive?" (For more on the anger circle and how it works, see Dr. Weisinger's *Anger Work Out Book*.)

betes did not mean that she was less of a person. She found that at last she could say "I have diabetes" without a trace of shame in her voice.

With this hurdle behind her, she was able to enjoy her social life again. Her friends respected her ability to control the disease and make difficult lifestyle changes to achieve better control.

Mary also used her feelings of anger to renew her closeness to her husband. When she began to feel angry, she would use the opportunity to talk to her husband. Instead of getting defensive about his concern, she learned to calm herself. When she felt in control, she made a point of telling him that she knew he was trying to help. She then explained why she was having a hard

Resources

The following books on anger may be available from your local library or bookstore:

Coping With Your Anger by Andrew D. Lester, Philadelphia: Westminster Press, 1983, paperback. Westminster Press, 925 Chesnut St., Philadelphia, PA 19107.

Overcoming Hurts and Anger by Dwight L. Carlson, MD, Eugene, OR.: Harvest House Publishers, 1981, paperback. Harvest House Publishers, 1075 Arrowsmith, Eugene, OR 97402.

Make Anger Your Ally by Neil Clark Warren, New York: Doubleday & Co., Inc., 1983, paperback.

Dr. Weisinger's Anger Work Out Book by Hendrie Weisinger, PhD, New York: William Morrow and Co., Inc., 1985, paperback. Wilmor Warehouse, 39 Plymouth St., P.O. Box 1219, Fairfield, NJ 07007.

time socializing. Together they agreed to let her have a little breathing room. She explained that one way he could show his support and acceptance of her diabetes was by coming to an ADA chapter meeting with her.

Let Anger Be Your Ally

The goal is not to eliminate anger from your life. You may continue to feel angry over the same issues. When you feel threatened, afraid, or frustrated, anger is an instinctive, protective response. But, as Mary discovered, you can learn to see your anger coming and put it to work for you. Mary's anger alerted her to the need for action. The better she understood her anger, the more she was able to use its power to help heal and resolve some of the conflicts in her everyday life.

Learning how to control and channel your anger takes time, commitment, and effort. Instead of putting a stranglehold on your diabetes care, anger can be your ally—a force for action, change, and growth.

Lorraine L. Cook, MSW, CCSW, *is a psychiatric social worker and psychotherapist in private practice in Ogden, Utah. She has had type 2 diabetes for 21 years and has been insulin-dependent for 8 years.*

16

Testing Your Attitude

by Robert M. Anderson and Robert W. Genthner

Who is responsible for your diabetes? Your attitude can make all the difference.

Diabetes, whether insulin-dependent or noninsulin-dependent, is a disease that requires a good deal of self-management.

To do that well, you have to understand whether your attitude toward having the disease helps you accept—or reject—responsibility for its care.

But it isn't always easy to realize what that attitude is. It's even more difficult to see how it can get in the way of good diabetes care.

That's why we drew up the PR—Personal Responsibility—scale. Originally, it was intended to help professionals understand the way patients look at their diabetes self-management.

We have adapted it here to help you evaluate your own self-management approach. It may also help you to recognize someone else's approach and to see how a change might lead to better diabetes control.

Of course, the scale doesn't begin to cover all the psychosocial issues associated with a chronic illness. It's only intended to give clues to your own attitude toward diabetes self-care.

Assumptions of the System

Let me begin by saying that the scale is based on three assumptions.

First, it assumes that human responsibility is a fact of life. As humans, we make choices. All choices have consequences. Therefore, we are responsible for the consequences of the choices we make.

Second, it assumes we can create meaning out of our own lives. Of course, we don't create all the circumstances of our lives—like having diabetes. But we give those circumstances their meaning.

For instance, some people see having diabetes as a disaster, while others view it as a challenge. The good news is that, since we put the meaning in the circumstances, we can also change that meaning when it seems to be hurting us.

Third, the system assumes that we are born with a drive to learn and to grow. We have to overcome many barriers before we fully realize our human potential. As we do, we move to higher levels of human growth.

How It Works

The PR scale has five levels, five being the most desirable. Knowing where you are on the scale can help you set your own goals for change.

Of course, everyone acts differently at different times, and no one will stay on the same level day in, day out. But certain attitudes and actions occur fairly regularly, and those are the ones on which to base your evaluations.

<u>Level 1:</u> People at this level take no responsibility for managing their own illness. They rarely accept the consequences of their actions, are uninterested in self-management, and seem overwhelmed by life.

In short, they act as if they are defeated victims who have given up.

Those at Level 1 spend the least amount of energy necessary to survive. They have little interest in caring—for themselves, even in their personal hygiene and grooming.

People here generally feel helpless in the face of diabetes, so they don't act with a specific goal in mind.

Curiously, people on Level 1 don't get angry easily, because they feel "it wouldn't do any good." In fact, when a person at Level 1 shows anger, it means he or she is moving to another level, because getting angry means beginning to fight back.

Because of their "I can't do it" attitude, people with diabetes who are at Level 1 are extremely dependent on relatives and medical professionals to manage their disease for them.

And because they feel they have no effect on anything, they'll say things like, "What's the use of following a diet? Nothing ever turns out right anyway." Or, simply, "Diabetes has ruined my life."

When you hear someone with diabetes say things like, "I can't learn it," "I can't do it," or "It's impossible to do everything I am supposed to do," you are probably talking to a person at Level 1.

<u>Level 2:</u> Here, some signs of personal responsibility are beginning to show up. People at Level 2 don't have

the defeated tone of those at Level 1, they are not willing to give up.

People at Level 2, however, may talk about their problems as though they belonged to someone else. They see outside forces as the cause of their difficulties. They make comments—like, "Diabetes changes the way people act," as if they were not personally involved.

Someone at Level 2 is either busy recovering from past struggles, or anticipating future problems.

Unlike people at Level 1 who are passive, people at Level 2 actively pursue the idea of themselves as victims. They blame outsiders so much that they even feel happiness comes from the outside, rather than from something they earned or caused.

Both those at Level 1 and Level 2 see themselves as victims. But, whereas those at Level 1 have given up, those at Level 2 use the victim approach to manipulate the world. They do believe they can change things, but only by getting others to do what they want.

Although people at Level 2 may feel some personal responsibility, they don't look for solutions within themselves. Instead, they fight back by getting angry, or by blaming others when things aren't going well. The fight against diabetes that people at Level 2 make is often aimed at others or at forces outside themselves, instead of at their own actions.

People here also often avoid a direct challenge, preferring to fight with backbiting and gossip. A person at Level 2 who develops ketoacidosis might blame the family, job, doctor, or hospital, instead of the way he or she handled diabetes. But, although they complain, they make no effort to change things at home or work or to file an official claim of poor care against the doctor or hospital.

Generally, someone at Level 2 is either busy recovering from past struggles or anticipating future problems. Those at this level rarely enjoy what they are doing at the moment, and any pleasure they gain from accomplishments usually comes from looking back at them.

There's a lot of self-pity on Level 2. People here may either complain or feel self-righteous because they are taking good care of themselves.

This self-pity also leads those at Level 2 to expect others to feel sorry for them. They might claim that no one understands how tough it is for them to handle their diabetes.

Because they blame others, the word "if" is common. "If only my wife cared about my diabetes, I'd be okay." "If only I didn't have such a bad memory, I would test my blood glucose more often." In other words, "If only other things were different, I'd be all right."

When you see someone spending a lot of energy finding others or outside causes to blame, feeling sorry for themselves, and not enjoying the moment, you probably are dealing with a person at Level 2.

<u>Level 3:</u> Here, people use their energy more productively than those at Level 2. Personal growth can occur at Level 3, because these people search for the difference between their own and other people's responsibility.

The difficulty comes because their focus, although starting out on themselves, often turns to others.

Although people at Level 3 might indeed be right about the wrongdoings of others, they use that knowledge to avoid recognizing their own involvement.

Someone at Level 3 might say, "I really should lose 20 pounds (admits own responsibility), but my wife always cooks fried foods (sees the fault in another and uses it)." They have a greater sense of fairness about the cause of their problems, but are still looking for someone else to share the blame.

This search for who is at fault makes people at Level

3 seem as though they are trying to be fair. But finding real faults in others, however correct, keeps one from examining his or her own role.

At this level, people tend to look closely at themselves only when things are going well.

You will hear someone at Level 3 using language that reflects this split between blaming others and taking responsibility. They use the words "You" or "one," but rarely "I."

For instance, "It's important to stay in good control when you have diabetes, but you rarely have time to test your blood glucose if you're a busy person." (No "I" words.)

Another favorite Level 3 word is "but." It points to the characteristic trait here—accepting responsibility, then shifting it to someone else. "I know I should talk to my doctor, but he's so difficult to reach."

<u>Level 4:</u> People at Level 4 talk about taking total responsibility for their lives. They look to themselves more than they do to others and rarely blame others for their unfortunate circumstances.

Although they accept responsibility, however, they don't always act on that acceptance.

People at Level 4 will say "I" often and understand that they should do things themselves. But they are short on the follow-through.

You might hear, "I need to lose weight and I know it's up to me. I just haven't done it." Or "I've been letting my control slip, and I need to improve."

People at Level 4 have a lot of energy, and are often into programs of physical, intellectual, or emotional growth. They focus more inward than outward and spend a minimum amount of time on the shortcomings of others. They don't dwell on the negative aspects of their illness, and don't spend time agonizing about complications that might occur in the future.

Moving to a higher level of PR will come naturally when you begin to talk over and solve your problems.

But, although they are aware, they don't always act.

Those at Level 4 view a crisis as a challenge. Yet, although they express confidence in their ability to respond successfully, it may not go much beyond that.

Although the person at Level 4 is close to maintaining good self-control of diabetes, he or she is still not quite there.

Taking responsibility for your diabetes, and listing good intentions are an excellent start. But they have to be carried out to be effective.

Level 5: At this level, people take total responsibility for their lives, and they act. They understand their own contribution to their well-being and know their own part when things don't go well.

Although they are capable of seeing reality and realize when others have not acted well, people at Level 5 don't dwell on how others may have contributed to their difficulties.

Here, people are operating at their peak most of the time. They have usually committed themselves to whatever effort is required to manage their diabetes. They act rather than waste resources or time in feeling sorry for themselves, blaming others, looking for excuses, or regretting mistakes.

At Level 5, people seldom give in to social pressures to drink or eat sweets because others are doing it.

When necessary, they make a decision and are not tormented by doubt over it. If they make a mistake, they use the information they gain to act differently next time.

People at Level 5 are fully aware of themselves, and are constantly finding ways to express increased personal responsibility. They examine their role in situations and use that knowledge to live healthier lives.

What may be a crisis for someone at another level is often an opportunity for growth here.

When people at Level 5 decide they need the resources of another person or a professional, they ask for help, but keep the responsibility for the outcome on themselves. They know it's up to them to make things work out.

At Level 5 you'll hear people talk mainly in straight-forward terms. "Since developing diabetes, I have a new way of understanding how my body uses food." Or, "Diabetes has helped me realize how much I value feeling well." They may also say, "Diabetes has made me more compassionate toward others."

Summary

If you notice that you are viewing your diabetes from a low level of personal responsibility, you are probably upset. You may feel criticized, unappreciated, or overwhelmed by all that you are supposed to do.

Don't blame yourself for being at a low level of PR. This will just make you feel worse. Instead, realize this is a good time to talk things over with someone you trust. Moving to a higher level of PR will come naturally when you begin to talk over and solve your problems.

The goal in diabetes self-management is to take responsibility for your own health care. Even if others have acted poorly or circumstances have not always worked out, it helps to know there is no profit in blaming others or looking outside yourself for solutions.

That's not an easy goal to reach, no matter what your age or diabetes regimen.

The PR system can give you a bit of insight into where you are on the road to that goal. It can help you and others see how strongly attitude affects diabetes care.

Robert Anderson, EdD, *is the associate director of the continuing education and outreach program at the University of Michigan Diabetes Research and Training Center in Ann Arbor.* **Robert Genthner** *is a clinical psychologist in private practice in Lexington, Kentucky.*

17

Starting a Support Group

Meeting with others who face the same problems can make all the difference.

by Kathryn Govaerts

Living with diabetes is not easy. Sometimes it can make you feel isolated or overwhelmed, and problems are compounded when you go away to college or start a new job. Although such changes are exciting, you may wonder how you'll meet the new challenges in your life and still manage your diabetes.

If you're moving to a new city or into a new living arrangement, you may also wonder how you'll keep your diabetes under control without the support of family and friends.

Good news! People in your community, or at your new college, work place, or city, can help. They—and you—have lots of wisdom to share. All you need is a way to get in touch.

While informal get-togethers are great ways to learn from each other, you'll probably find even greater benefits from more formalized contacts. Where do you find those kinds of contacts? In a support group.

What to Expect

Groups for people with shared concerns are not new. Since the first known medical support group was founded in 1905 (the members all had tuberculosis), the idea has taken root and flourished.

A support group is an established, ongoing meeting of people who have common concerns, goals, and interests. It fosters the notion that each member's feelings, ideas, fears, and hopes are probably not the exception; in fact, they are often the rule.

A support group is geared toward the specific needs of its members. Many people find that meeting together encourages group as well as individual problem solving.

If you join a group, you'll probably find that listening to others will bring new ideas and insights into your own situation, some of which you may translate into new behaviors.

What's more, you will be giving your thoughts to others. They may then put your ideas into practice, or find that your support, understanding, or idea helps them cope a little better, too. That not only helps them, it can give you new confidence and a feeling of accomplishment.

A support group does not have to be set up to run for a long period of time. It can be time-limited, meeting only a few sessions to carry out a specific agenda and goal. Or, it may continue for an extended period, perhaps months or even years, with different members entering and leaving as their situations dictate.

What a Support Group Is Not

While it is good to understand what a support group is, it is equally important to know what it is not.

Support groups are not psychotherapy groups. People who join a psychotherapy group are going through fairly significant levels of emotional distress.

Leaders of these groups require training in psychotherapeutic techniques. They are responsible for selecting group participants and for keeping group focus and goals clear.

In a psychotherapy group, you must be an active participant and attend regularly to get the maximum value out of the group.

Furthermore, you generally pay—often a rather substantial sum—when the group is run by a professional. That is appropriate if you need professional help.

However, when you join a group of people who are getting together without a professional therapist, there is usually little or no money changing hands.

Getting Ready

Let's assume you are eager for contact with others who have diabetes, but do not need the services of a professional psychotherapist.

The group you want to be in may be for people who have type 1 (insulin-dependent), type 2 (non-insulin-dependent) diabetes, either type, or for those who care for someone with diabetes. It may be for people in a certain age range, or those living in one community.

For instance, your group might be composed of students at a particular university who have insulin-dependent diabetes, or adults with non-insulin-dependent diabetes who work in the same company or live in the same community. It may even consist of parents with children who have type 1 diabetes, or of people on an insulin pump.

After you have decided its composition, determine if such a group already exists in your area. Call your local American Diabetes Association, area diabetologists, and mental health professionals. Don't forget to ask the administration office of your university or company if such a group is registered. (These groups register so they can use the facilities.)

Also check calendars of events in local newspapers and hospitals to see if a similar group is already meeting.

If you don't locate a group, start one yourself. However, it's important to understand that no group can meet all the needs and wants of all of its members all of the time.

Unlike a group that meets under the professional eye of a psychotherapist, the group you form will make democratic decisions about meeting times, places, length the group will continue, how to maintain itself, and rules it should function by.

Forming Your Group

To form a successful group, it's essential to locate people who fit your criteria. Be systematic about your inquiry.

Request information from student and employee health centers, area physicians and diabetes educators, as well as mental health and employee assistance counselors.

Your local ADA chapter can help. Ask your chapter, as well as local hospitals and community clinics, to sponsor you by telling interested people how to get in touch with your newly formed group.

Once you locate potential members, find out their interests. Set up an information sheet with names, addresses, and phone numbers of possible members, and a short list of reasons they want to join.

If you find interested people (and most likely you will), your next step is to plan the first meeting.

Step 1. Choose the date. Review the community, school, organization, or company calendar to select a free date. Also, look at city events and the local high school and professional sports calendar.

You don't want your first meeting to conflict with a popular event. Even the most eager members will find it difficult to attend in the middle of exams, or when they have tickets for the theater.

Step 2. Find a meeting place. After you pick the date, look for an appropriate place, preferably where you can meet free of charge. A school might allow you to use a classroom. Libraries often have meeting rooms for neighborhood gatherings, as do churches and synagogues. Ask at a local hospital. If this is a companywide organization or university group, call the administration office and ask for the use of a room.

Step 3. Plan the first meeting. It is essential to plan the first meeting exceptionally well. Choose a dynamic speaker on a topic that has broad appeal, one you identified in your initial survey as being of general interest. Have a brief agenda of items that need to be discussed, like meeting times, etc.

Step 4. Get the word out. Advertise your meeting in neighborhood newspapers, company or school newsletters, even in supermarkets. Start at least four weeks in advance.

Ask people to announce the meeting in clubs, bingo parlors, and so on. Request an announcement to be made in churches and synagogues.

Don't forget word of mouth. Friend telling friend is often the best way to get a crowd. Ask each person to phone one other likely candidate.

Try to reach as many people as possible, especially within the interests and age framework you have established. But don't worry that you are reaching people who do not have diabetes, also. They may have friends, children, or other family members looking for just such a group.

<u>Step 5.</u> Send reminders. A week to 10 days before the meeting, send reminder cards or make phone calls to keep interest high.

Meeting Called to Order

At the first get together, let everyone participate in setting a regular day, time, and place for future meetings—say the first Saturday or second Tuesday of the month. That will help make meetings part of everyone's regular schedule.

Although there may be a great deal of enthusiasm at the first gathering, don't have meetings close together. Generally, getting together once a week will burn people out quickly. Every other week is better, and many groups meet once a month.

Consider less traditional meeting times, too. You might pick a Saturday morning, breakfast hour, or lunchtime, if everyone is in the same school or company. This could be especially helpful if people are concerned about being out after dark.

No matter when you meet, be sure to begin and end on time so members can count on how long they will be there. This not only helps plan meetings, but lets participants know their time and attendance are not treated lightly.

If your first agenda calls for selecting officers or even committees (perhaps a program committee and a telephone reminder committee), it's a good idea to have a few people ready to "volunteer." Their enthusiasm will be contagious.

Agendas will vary. Some groups may want most of their meetings focused on gathering information on diabetes care. Others may want speakers on relevant, but not necessarily medical topics, such as career information when you have diabetes, finding appropriate insurance, or advances in diabetes research.

To find speakers and subjects, tap area sources like student or employee health personnel, mental health professionals, physicians, diabetes educators, nurses, exercise specialists, and the local chapter of the American Diabetes Association.

Be sure to leave time for discussion.

Extras

Many groups have a social period after the regular meeting. You might make the meeting an hour and a half, then have a half-hour social time.

If the group votes for it, you could have soft drinks, coffee, sandwiches, or snacks at the social. If you are meeting in a company or organization building, they may have a coffee maker to lend you.

Serving food means that people will either have to donate the goodies—perhaps on a rotating schedule—give a small amount of money, if they can afford it. (Don't assume they can.) It's possible that a local organization or business—say, a supermarket—might donate snacks.

You could even work the foods into the meeting, with everyone figuring out the Exchanges based on the American Diabetes Association/The American Dietetic Association's *Exchange Lists for Meal Planning.*

Remember that only appropriate food should be served, avoiding saturated fats as well as sweets.

Depending on the group, it might be a good idea to hire a baby-sitter for the meeting period. Or, perhaps a family member could volunteer. For those who have small children, this could make the difference between attending or staying home.

Pitfalls

Certain pitfalls can be the death knell of the group. If most of the time is spent in pessimistic complaining without active problem solving, all but the complainers will quickly lose interest.

Be aware of the person who monopolizes the talk and has an agenda that is only of interest to a few members.

Cliques tend to create tension and will discourage new members from committing to the group's goals. Unresolved conflicts and rivalry between individuals and sub-groups are detrimental and should be avoided or stopped as soon as they start.

Give all interested people the chance to plan meetings and work with as many members as possible.

That will build cohesiveness and counter a splintering effect. Let people know that everyone with something constructive to say will have time to speak. Don't stifle one person to give another time. Make sure people listen when someone is talking.

Groups have a natural life span. If attendance at meetings lessens, then enthusiasm wanes and a few are left carrying the responsibility for all. When this happens it's likely the usefulness of the group needs to be reevaluated.

Keeping the Group Going

Groups require a certain degree of nurturing to keep them alive. Ask people to sign their names to a list at each meeting so you will know those members who come regularly and those who drop out. Notice whether the membership is growing or declining.

When new people come in, be sure to make them feel welcome and valued. Get their names and introduce them. Consider name tags if the group numbers over 15 or so.

You may find that the focus of the group changes over time. What started out to be an information sharing group may become focused on activities instead. If this meets the needs of the majority of the membership, such changes are acceptable.

Saying Goodbye

If the group agreed to meet for a specific length of time—say one semester or until an activity is completed—its ending is easier.

It's possible that another series of meetings will be agreed to, or another project begun. It's also possible that the group will have met its original goals and that it is indeed time to say goodbye.

Specific closing activities and messages are important so that members leave with a sense of satisfaction and closure. It is helpful to review the original goals and point out those that were met and those that were not. (If the group has gone on for some time, you may find that the membership, as well as the way meetings are conducted, have changed quite a bit.)

Any outstanding bills must be paid, of course, and, you or the group must return borrowed supplies or equipment. Be sure to notify sponsoring agencies not to send further referrals. Finally, notify the building where you are meeting that you will no longer need the room.

As you run through the final tasks of winding up your support group, you're likely to agree that meeting

With A Little Support, We Can Cope

The first thing we thought of when our daughter Leata was diagnosed with diabetes was getting help for her. But as parents, we also struggled with the impact of the illness. Although the doctors and nurses assured us we were handling it well, that did not seem like enough.

In those first months, diabetes overshadowed everything. Preparing Exchange-calculated meals, going to my daughter's elementary school to check her blood sugar, often making a second trip in response to an overreacting teacher, not wanting to discourage her concern, all left little time for anything else.

There were other problems. What to do about the little boy in class who told everyone they would catch what my daughter had if they played with her? Should I drive her to school to make her feel protected, or let her walk and agonize about what might happen on the way?

I knew talking to a professional counselor would help, but the person I really wanted to talk to was the parent of another child with diabetes.

The first such parent I found was a mother whose daughter had been diagnosed before her second birthday. I dialed her number with a lot of expectations, but diabetes had taken a toll on the family, and I could get no help from them.

Finally, I called my local American Diabetes Association chapter. We found that other parents had already started a support group that had become inactive. With the help of the chapter, and the other parents, we reactivated that original Parent-Youth Diabetes Support Group of San Mateo County, Calif.

We started up again with five families, and now, five years later, we have 40. In fact, we will probably split into two groups soon, with one for teenagers.

No one was sure what format to use at the first meeting of the reactivated group, but somehow we simply talked and talked until the janitor wanted the room.

A format did evolve, and today we hold simultaneous meetings in separate rooms for parents and children. The kids have an older teenager in charge. Sometimes they compare meters or talk about giving injections or see a videotape on camps for children with diabetes. Mostly they make a lot of noise and enjoy each other—normal kids who happen to have diabetes.

We are particularly good with families of newly diagnosed children. As Carol Harris, current Executive Director of the San Mateo County Chapter of the ADA, put it, "The group just embraces the new family, and lets them know they are not handling this alone."

Often, we have a health professional speak to us, then answer questions. The heart of the meetings, however, is simply people sharing experiences, wisdom, and sometimes pain, with others who understand.

Need a baby-sitter? Want to find sugar-free Valentine's Day candy? Someone in the group will know. Not all problems have easy answers, but we can always talk about them.

When the mother of a newly diagnosed girl told us their doctor said urine testing was adequate, we responded in a chorus, "Change doctors."

A father was showing the strain of dealing with his 14-year-old son who would not stick to his food plan. At first, the group could offer little but understanding. Most of us had experienced a child's rebellion. Then someone asked what the boy's food plan was. When the father said "1200 calories," we could indeed offer more than sympathy—we could offer a list of dietitians who would supply what we knew was a reasonable calorie count for his son.

After five years in the support group, our family knows a lot. Counting exchanges comes easy now and my daughter does her own testing and injecting. She packs her diabetes supplies more easily than her toothbrush when she heads for an overnight. She's lost a coat, three pairs of shoes, and innumerable sweaters. But she's never lost her blood-glucose monitor. She's been to camp for two summers and gained great confidence there.

We can share her success—and ours—with others in the group. And we will look to them when we face new challenges, like the teen years, dating, and driving. With a little support, I know we can cope.

—Jan Holloway, Montara, California

The Minority Adult Support Group of St. Louis

Robert Shornick of St. Louis, Mo., has insulin-dependent diabetes, and several years ago he and his wife, Betty, began an adult support group for the St. Louis chapter of the American Diabetes Association. But the Shornicks noticed that the group had only about a 10 percent minority membership.

Bob and Betty felt that a support group in another location might make it more accessible to the city's minority population.

"We decided that for minorities to attend, the group had to be where they are, in the inner city," Robert explains.

So, in August 1989, Robert and Betty, with help from Gerri Phelps, RN, community services director at Regional Hospital in St. Louis, started the Minority Adult Support Group in the St. Louis inner city. The group is under the sponsorship of the St. Louis Chapter of the American Diabetes Association, which provides the funds.

The St. Louis Regional Hospital, where the group meets, provides the facility.

"We have about 50 to 60 people at each meeting," Gerri says, "and, though we are mainly from minorities, everyone feels welcome. We are very supportive of one another."

Betty Shornick recalls the group's beginnings two years ago. "We knocked on as many doors and made as many calls as we could," she says. The Shornicks still write notices to inner-city ministers, advertise in minority newspapers, request radio announcements, and print notices, and they mail out reminders. Betty even makes personal calls to members each month. "All newcomers are welcomed with genuine warmth," says Robert, who adds, "And we have fun, too."

The group gathers the last Saturday morning each month for a one-and-one-half hour program, followed by a social. "We continue talking over sandwiches, coffee, and soft drinks," Robert says. The group also provides free child care for attendees.

Anyone who wants to speak during the meetings gets a chance. The only rule is that when one person is talking, everyone else must listen.

Subjects include a variety of areas such as exercise, stress, family relations, communicating with doctors, diet, and food exchanges. American Diabetes Association booklets are distributed.

"When people share experiences, they find that others have survived the same problems. Then we all have a new sense of self-esteem," Robert sums up. Although the group has expanded, the Shornicks explain, "it's easy to start a support group, difficult to keep it going, and almost impossible to make it grow."

In April, the Shornicks retired as leaders. Now Gerri Phelps, Karen Bass, and Gladys Rose, all connected with Regional Hospital, will keep the group going. "It's been a wonderful program for people with diabetes in the inner city," Gerri concludes.

with people who understand and empathize with your particular situation can be very valuable and satisfying.

Diabetes management can definitely be a lot easier with a little help from your friends.

***

Kathryn Govaerts, PhD, *is in private practice in pediatric psychology in Tulsa, Oklahoma.*

Part II:
If You Really Want to Help…

18
A Willing Heart…

...is half the battle. But when you want to help someone you care about who has diabetes, you've got to know how.

by Janet Meirelles

Y ou want to be as helpful as possible to family members or friends who have diabetes. That's great. But sometimes good intentions don't work out as planned.

Kindness doesn't always light the way, either. For instance, it seems kind to help a friend forget diabetes for a few hours, or to encourage him or her to enjoy all the foods everyone else is digging into "just this once." But such an approach may do more harm than good.

Perhaps the best way to help people with diabetes is to allow them to stick to the basic rule of good diabetes care. The rule is simple, and it applies to those with type 1 (insulin-dependent) and type 2 (non-insulin-dependent) diabetes: Take control of your own life.

If you're not sure that's the approach you always take and if you have the courage to indulge in a bit of self-reflection, see if you recognize yourself in this list of hopeful helpfuls.

The Hopeful Helpfuls

The Pusher

You want your dinner guests to relax, enjoy themselves, and eat all the wonderful food you've prepared. You certainly don't want anyone to pass up your special main dish or dessert.

But there sits your best friend, niece, nephew, or grandchild turning down second helpings, or refusing your homemade cake. It doesn't seem right. Why shouldn't someone with diabetes have as good a time as everyone else?

So you plead, "I made it just for you," or, "You'll hurt my feelings if you don't eat it." After all, you only want them to enjoy themselves.

You've got a point, of course. All people should enjoy themselves at a happy gathering. But eating something that's heavy on the fat or sugar is not the only—or even the best—way to do that. And the cake that tastes so good now will seem far less inviting later when it elevates the blood glucose of someone you care about.

More important: When you make someone with diabetes give in to your requests, you help break down that person's self-discipline. That means that when you win, the person with diabetes loses.

Even though you mean well, twisting people's arms to get them to do what you want them to do is counterproductive: Such coercion just eats away at their self-control.

The Protector

You are a warm hearted person, and you don't want anyone you care about who has diabetes to do anything you think harmful.

In fact, you're so concerned that, no matter what the person's age, you blur the line between that individual's responsibility for his or her own health care and yours. So you become a protector.

That leads you to make remarks such as, "Put on a sweater. Remember your diabetes," or, "You shouldn't be eating that cake even if it is your birthday," or even, "Don't walk too far. You have diabetes, you know."

Relax. Having diabetes doesn't mean people have to bundle up as if they were ill. Birthday celebrants with diabetes can even have a piece of birthday cake—if they plan ahead for it. That's what the American Diabetes Association, The American Dietetic Association Exchange Lists for Meal Planning are all about. They help people with diabetes "exchange" one food for another.

Having diabetes doesn't mean one has to haul out the car for every errand either. Exercise is not just permitted; it's an important part of the diabetes regimen, and walking instead of driving is a fine way to exercise.

But the real danger in being a protector is that your protection can backfire. If it works, it can make the person with diabetes dependent on you, which is not a good way to handle the disease.

Or, human nature being what it is, it can make someone who gets a lot of advice turn rebellious.

Like the pusher, your best bet is to focus on what people with diabetes need most: the chance to take control of their own lives.

The Advertiser

"Let me introduce you to Joan. We have to be careful about what we serve her. She's a diabetic."

"Will everyone in the audience who is diabetic please raise his or her hand for a minute?"

If you see nothing wrong with those two phrases, you may be an advertiser.

That means that, first, you may be denying someone's individuality by labeling him or her "a diabetic." Not everyone with diabetes appreciates being identified by the disease. For instance, Joan might prefer to be introduced as an insurance adjuster, a New Englander, or a hockey fan, rather than "a diabetic."

Second, by telling Joan's new acquaintance that Joan has diabetes, or by asking anyone with the disease to state the fact in public, you are robbing people of their personal privacy. There are probably few of us who would like everyone we meet to know the status of our health.

(Certainly, someone at this function should be aware that Joan has diabetes in case she needs help, but it's up to Joan to decide who that someone should be.)

"But," you may be wondering, "what if I have a reason to talk about someone's diabetes? Maybe I want to introduce two people and let them know they both have the same disease." It's still a good idea to ask, in private, if either would mind if you mentioned it.

Look at it this way. You wouldn't open a door in someone's home without knocking on it first. So why open the door to the status of someone's health without asking?

The Analyzer

You probably know that a very low blood glucose level—called an insulin reaction—can lead people to act irritable and cranky. And you know that an insulin reaction is serious and requires quick treatment with glucose or something sugary.

So, at the mere suggestion of crankiness in a friend who is taking insulin, you tell him or her, "You must be having an insulin reaction. You better drink some orange juice or take your glucose."

What's wrong with that?

For one, you're presuming a lot. Maybe your friend's crankiness has nothing to do with diabetes. After all, people who don't have diabetes get irritated, too. So begin by asking the same question you'd ask anybody else who appeared agitated: "Is anything wrong?"

Remember, no one likes to be analyzed, treated as if they didn't know their own needs, and told what to do, even though an insulin reaction can blur one's thinking.

This is not to say that you should ignore sudden changes in your friend's behavior. But, by all means, attempt to come to a mutual understanding beforehand. You might find things work out more smoothly if you discuss the matter with your friend when you are both calm. Ask if he or she wants you to sound an alert when you think something isn't right.

If your friend agrees, then even if you get rebuffed, you have been granted permission to mention, even to pursue, the idea that he or she might be in some difficulty.

But it's still a delicate matter.

There is another good reason for handling the matter judiciously. Your pronouncement—"You must be having an insulin reaction" could cause your friend, who is already irritated, to say, "No, I'm not," or, "I can handle it," even if he or she does need to take a blood glucose reading—and would have done so if left alone.

The Ignorer

"We're all going out for drinks and then on to dinner somewhere. Come on. Don't be a party pooper."

Is that you on Friday after work? If so, and there is someone with either type 1 or type 2 diabetes in the crowd, you might not realize it, but you could be labeled an ignorer.

While that seems like a good thing—after all, it's the opposite of the advertiser—it can have unintended consequences.

That isn't your intention, of course. You only want to help your friend forget everything, including diabetes, for a couple of hours. But checking your plans with the member of the party who has diabetes would be a useful courtesy.

For one thing, alcohol, when consumed without food, can play havoc with blood glucose levels.

Another point: People who are taking insulin have to stay on a well defined eating schedule. They also have to know when to inject the insulin. Usually, that's done about 15 to 45 minutes before eating. That means they need a definite and secure dinner time.

So, despite your good intentions, as an ignorer you may be arranging for your friend with diabetes to take unnecessary health risks.

Certainly people with diabetes know how to care for themselves at get-togethers. But you can make life easier by asking quietly what plans would help them stay on their diabetes schedule.

The Worrier

Your mom, dad, grandma, or granddad had diabetes and didn't fare too well. Perhaps one of them had a foot amputated, developed eye trouble, or died young from a heart attack.

So whenever you meet people with diabetes, you let them know what a serious disease it is, that they should be careful and expect trouble.

Of course, if you are a regular *Diabetes Forecast* reader, you know about the revolution in diabetes care since your parents' time.

When you make someone with diabetes give in to your requests, you help break down that person's self-discipline.

But if you are reading this book for the first time in a doctor's office or someone's home, be assured that diabetes treatment has come a very long way in just a few years.

Self-monitoring of blood glucose allows people with diabetes to test their own blood glucose levels any time of the day or night. They can then adjust the amount of insulin or medication they take, the quantity of food they eat, or the level of exercise they engage in, if necessary.

There are also sophisticated laser treatments for eye difficulties, and insulins with very few impurities to help prevent insulin allergies. Even kidney and pancreas transplants are not uncommon.

You should certainly know about the Diabetes Complications and Control Trial (DCCT), the most comprehensive study of diabetes control ever. It asked the question: Can tight blood glucose control (keeping blood glucose levels close to the norm) help prevent or delay complications in people with type 1 diabetes. The answer? Yes, it definitely can.

So, if you're a worrier, feel free to put some of your concerns to rest.

Diabetes research is continuing to bring us easier, more effective ways to deal with this disease. And you can be assured that your parents' or grandparents' experiences with diabetes are far from the norm today.

Help, Don't Hurt

Of course, all of the above traps have their origin in caring. You're eager to help, and that's commendable. Unfortunately, that isn't always enough.

The desire to be useful brings its own obligation: simply to couple a knowledgeable mind to a kind and loving heart.

Janet Meirelles, RN, CDE, *is in private practice in Lake Oswego, Oregon. She is also co-chair of the Oregon Diabetes Educators Professional Education Committee. Her book,* Diabetes Is Not A Piece of Cake, *written for families and friends of people with diabetes, was published in 1994.*

19
Six Secrets of Successful Parenting

No one ever said that coping with a child's diabetes was easy, but many families find a way to take it in stride.

by Debbie Lloyd

Your child has just been diagnosed with diabetes. You can hardly believe that injections, blood tests, and meal schedules will be part of your little girl's or boy's life—and yours—from now on.

Like all parents, you are working through a sense of shock as well as a restructuring of family priorities.

Virtually all parents whose children are diagnosed with a chronic illness go through this emotional whirlwind. Some recover quickly and become the able caregivers that a young child with a chronic disease requires. But others find it a constant strain.

What is it that helps successful parents adjust?

Over the years I've studied families that have taken diabetes in stride. Based on their experiences, I've put together six characteristics that seem to make a difference.

Six Ways Parents Succeed

1. Deal With Their Own Emotions

The emotional factor is the largest barrier that prevents parents from handling a child's diagnosis well. And no wonder. Often parents have to get past an array of negative feelings. Perhaps they feel that the diabetes could have been prevented or that some of the fault lies with them.

And certainly they have to work through a changed perception of their world. Where once they faced a cloudless future for their child, they now see problems and uncertainty.

They also have to deal with the fact that their child's life—and their family's—will never be as carefree as it was before the diagnosis.

It's clear that parents who cope well with these issues soon learn to drop the "if onlys." They don't categorize their presumed failures or dwell on what might have been.

It's not that they don't have such thoughts. Of course, they do. But they don't focus on them. Certainly they are aware of the possibility of complications down the line. But they understand that they play a real part in making their child as healthy as possible both today and tomorrow. And that helps them stick with their primary goal, coping with the needs of today.

2. Handle Their Child's Distress

Certainly no parent wants to cause his or her child pain. But parents whose son or daughter has diabetes face a dilemma. Giving injections, testing blood glucose, or denying a plea for a candy bar does give a child pain. Yet a child needs this pain to maintain good health.

Parents who cope well handle this dilemma by separating their daughter's or son's immediate discomfort from the long view of a healthy diabetes regimen.

Sure it's tough to hear your girl or boy scream, "I hate my finger stick," or even "I hate you." And the easiest course is for a mom or dad to say, "OK, we'll skip it this once," or "Go ahead and eat a small piece. I don't suppose it can hurt. Just stop crying."

But wise parents know that the best thing they can do for their youngster is to be strong themselves. They continue the necessary procedures, calmly and gently, but firmly—either they understand instinctively, or have been counseled that their own strength and consistency actually make it easier for their child to handle the diabetes regimen.

Look at it this way. If the parent is strong and consistent, the child doesn't have to go through tears and tantrums each time something unpleasant comes up, because those tears and tantrums never work.

On the other hand, if they sometimes work, a child with any gumption at all will keep trying them. So the best thing a parent can do is show a child that the test or the injection is inevitable, and that the best course is to accept it and move on.

It's tough for a parent to bring a child to that point. But parents who cope well finally accept the fact that they must cause their child brief pain today in order to keep him or her in good health tomorrow. And they don't rethink that decision every time something painful needs to be done.

However, these parents also know that it helps to let the child express anger at the injection or test. In fact, it brings a kind of closeness if all agree that diabetes is not fair. If the child is very young, a parent and child may even stamp around the house together, announcing, "I hate diabetes." Allowing a child to be angry at the disease may actually help a youngster accept the regimen.

3. Learn to "Partialize"

It's easy to feel overwhelmed when you are bombarded by a multitude of emotions as well as a list of new and sometimes difficult tasks. Some parents learn to handle all this through a system I call "partializing."

That means they take each part of their child's diabetes care separately, instead of struggling under the full weight of the diabetes diagnosis and detailed regimen.

For instance, they don't go over and over a seemingly unending list of chores. "We've got to figure out what foods to buy, and how to have a healthy meal every morning, noon, and evening while deciding how to administer blood glucose tests and insulin injections, and, oh yes, figure out whether to tell the neighbors and Aunt Sarah that Chris has diabetes, and who is going to go to the doctor for all the appointments, and should we take that vacation next month or stay home?"

Anyone would be overwhelmed by such a list. But parents who cope well divide the duties and concerns.

First, they parcel out their child's needs between them, and include extended family if they are available and capable. After all, there is no law that says only the mother can prepare meals, or only the father can check on the child during the night, or that grandma can't learn about diabetes care and take her grandchild for a weekend.

Second, they "partialize" their individual schedules. Everything needn't be a continuous stream of worries. Some things, such as injections and tests, do need immediate attention. But others, even grocery lists, can wait a bit. Certainly next month's vacation or a birthday party six months down the road is not a high priority.

The Chinese have a saying: The longest trip begins with a single step. And the most complex diabetes care begins with simple steps, too, something that successful parents seem to learn fairly quickly.

4. Remember Their Own Needs

Curiously, parents who cope well with a child's diabetes don't dwell exclusively on the child's difficulties or the diabetes.

They maintain meaningful relationships with other adults, keep their houses pleasant and attractive, and enjoy a job, hobby, friends, and evenings away from the child.

These moms and dads have a strong sense of their inner selves, an awareness of their own needs as well as their child's. They know that it's not enough to keep their child in good physical and mental health. They must keep themselves that way, too.

Sometimes these parents have a ready-made support system to lean on. It might be family, friends, or a particularly trusted and friendly health care team. Others get that help from support groups composed of other parents of children with diabetes.

And if these self-aware parents find themselves having emotional difficulties because of their child's diagnosis, they have no problem seeking professional help for themselves.

After all, there is nothing noble about neglecting oneself or being a martyr, yet it's easy to fall into that role when you have a child with diabetes. Wise moms and dads learn not to fall into that pit, or they crawl out of it quickly if they do.

5. Accept the Food Challenge

Food presents a real challenge to parents dealing with a child who has diabetes. To succeed with any part of

Virtually all parents whose children are diagnosed with a chronic illness go through this emotional whirlwind.

the diabetes regimen, they have to cope well with this area of their child's and their family's life.

It's clear that certain tips help. For instance, they give their child a choice of foods rather than a command to "eat this." And you will hear them say things such as, "You can have either milk and cereal or cheese and crackers for your snack. Which would you like?"

That kind of choice gives the child a sense of control, which seems to make most children calmer and more open to other requests.

Parents also do well when they keep the mealtime atmosphere pleasant and light. They don't turn dinnertime into discipline time. Rather, they show their child that food is to be enjoyed.

It's surprising how quickly children learn to model their table behavior after their parents. In fact, when you see a child who is comfortable and pleasant while eating away from home, you can be sure the parents do a good job handling mealtimes.

But there's another difficulty concerning food. This involves parents who have at least one child with diabetes and one or more others who do not. Should the children eat different foods at meals?

The best answer seems to be "no." The whole family should have the same menu. After all, the diabetes diet is healthy for everyone. And today's kids, whether they have any special medical concerns or not, are tuned into health and nutrition at school and even on the TV.

Eating the same meals also helps maintain a sense of unity within the entire family.

6. Accept the Diagnosis

Finally, successful parents learn to accept the diagnosis and move on. In fact, there is no "moving on" if they do not accept the reality of their child's diabetes.

Parents do well when they keep the mealtime atmosphere pleasant and light.

Yet acceptance doesn't happen at once. It's a process that may take weeks, months, even years. And even after parents do accept the diagnosis, it's not unusual for them occasionally to slip back into the sadness and frustration they felt during the first weeks.

But parents work hard to accept the diabetes because they see how their own attitude helps their child.

Young children are sensitive to their parents' emotional states. If mom or dad continues to feel unfairly treated by fate, or put upon by the diabetes regimen, the child will pick that up. He or she may then feel a sense of guilt for bringing all this unhappiness on the family. The child will probably also feel cheated and put upon, too.

No matter how they are feeling about the diagnosis themselves, successful parents grasp the fact that diabetes will be part of their children's and their own lives from now on, and that their family will be better off if it works with the disease rather than against it.

Finally, it's important for parents of newly diagnosed children to know what great resiliency they have. Most parents show remarkable ability to meet the challenges a child's diabetes diagnosis brings. Acceptance may not come at once, but it does come.

They achieve a well-balanced lifestyle, not only for their child, but for themselves as well. Actually, despite all they have to face, most parents handle things extremely well. And that's a joy to see.

Debbie Lloyd, MSW, *is a child and family therapist at InterCare Options in Pittsburgh, Pennsylvania.*

20

"Mommy, I Don't Want to Be Different"

Although diabetes affects children physically, it needn't harm their spirits.

by Peggy Finston

Any chronic illness will make a child—whether 5 or 15—feel different from other kids, both in the child's own eyes and in the eyes of friends. But feeling "different" may also make a child feel uncomfortable, hurt, or even cheated.

Parents often try to console their children with diabetes with lines such as, "No one's perfect," and "Wouldn't it be a boring world if everyone were the same?"

Though true, these statements don't address the heart of the problem: the anger, hurt, and sense of deprivation that children with chronic illnesses feel.

What About a Child With Diabetes?

It's not unusual for a child with a chronic illness to vacillate between feeling special and feeling upset.

Although children with diabetes don't look or act any different from their peers, that doesn't mean that they escape the uncomfortable special attention that a chronic illness can bring. Friends still observe kids with diabetes checking their blood glucose levels, taking insulin, snacking and eating at special times, and choosing foods with great care.

The youngster with diabetes also has special worries. Do the other kids know I have diabetes? If they know, what do they think of me? If they don't know, should I tell them?

Most important, just because differences are invisible does not mean they grant the child immunity from feeling anxious or uncomfortable.

Here's Help

Psychiatrists and other mental health professionals have found ways for parents to help a child handle the emotional side of diabetes and maintain a positive sense of self. Here is an extensive list of suggestions that may help.

* Start talking to your child early about his or her diabetes, and communicate more than just the facts. Make your manner and tone matter-of-fact. Don't convey pity. "You poor kid. Look what you got stuck with," doesn't help. However, do listen empathetically when your child speaks to you about his or her feelings.
* Don't place blame. Stay away from lines such as, "It's too bad you had to get this, but daddy's (or mommy's) mother had it and I guess you got it from her."
* Listen to your child. Stay tuned for indications that he or she doesn't fully understand the illness. Be alert to clues that tell you how your youngster feels about diabetes, and why.

For example, your child may see diabetes as a punishment. ("I was mean to my little brother and that's why I got it.") Or, your child may avoid old friends because he or she thinks that diabetes is contagious.

* Be prepared for a child's contradictory feelings. When 12-year-old Todd was in the hospital, his friends came to visit. Todd proudly showed them how brave he was by doing his blood glucose tests and giving himself insulin injections in front of them.

But when his friends left, Todd ripped off his medical identification bracelet because it said to him that he was different, with a difference he didn't like.

It's not unusual for a youngster with a chronic illness to vacillate between feeling special and feeling upset. So, congratulate your child on his or her courage and competence in handling the disease, but let your youngster blow off steam, too.

* Be a listener, not a constant advisor. Well-meaning, but routine reassurances, such as, "Diabetes isn't going to hurt your life," may inadvertently stop your child from talking further with you about the way he or she feels.

Sometimes kids—like the rest of us—just want to bounce ideas off someone else, or solve problems by themselves.

* Let your youngster practice talking to you about diabetes. That, in turn, will make it easier for him or her to discuss the illness with others. And when you and your child are with others, make sure it is the child, not you, who does any talking about diabetes. The last thing you want is to become a spokesperson for your child. That only undermines his or her mastery and sense of control over the illness.

When practicing, keep in mind that a child's explanation to friends can be very simple. "I have diabetes. That means my body doesn't use sugar the way yours does." As your child gets older, he or she will understand more and will be able to explain more about it—if he or she wants to do so.

* Consider humor. A smile can ease the tension, even when something serious is being discussed. I heard one 8-year-old describe his snacks as "a glucose recharge."
* Let your child know that, although there's nothing wrong with talking about diabetes, he or she does not owe anyone an explanation of it.

An injection or snack can rob children of privacy. Even so, the choice not to talk about the reason for the snack or the injection remains theirs. (Of course, teachers, athletic coaches, school medical personnel, and the like should know your child has diabetes, and understand appropriate responses to an insulin reaction.)

* If your child wants your help in dealing with friends, you might give him or her an insulin injection in front of the friends, or let them hold some of the diabetes equipment. (However, as a health measure, do not test other children's blood glucose.) Making your child's friends comfortable with diabetes is not your responsibility. Still, putting them at ease with the illness may help your child be at ease with it, too.
* Ask if your child wants to have a classroom session on diabetes. (Often a teacher has as little knowledge of this condition as the children.)

If the child is interested (but only then), contact the teacher and ask if you can set up a session on diabetes. You might do the talking yourself, if that makes your child more comfortable, or attend as a backup for your child, who will give the presentation.

When 9-year-old Brenda realized her classmates were questioning her about her snacks, she agreed to have her mother talk about diabetes to them.

Brenda's mom first assured everyone that diabetes was not contagious, a common unspoken fear of children.

Then she explained that Brenda's body did not use food the way everyone else's did. She showed them the insulin bottle and syringe and explained insulin as a kind of wonder drug that helped Brenda's body use food correctly.

She also told them that, because Brenda took insulin before she came to school, she needed a morning snack for the insulin to act on.

Brenda's mom also pointed out how brave Brenda was to test her blood glucose and give herself (or receive) insulin injections several times a day.

* Help your child interpret the way others respond to diabetes.

If your child is sensitive, he or she may feel hurt by any remark that draws attention to the diabetes. Even a simple, "Why do you eat special foods?" may seem unkind. Help him or her distinguish curiosity from meanness.

On the other hand, if your child feels teased or taunted, listen to the feelings he or she expresses. If necessary, help your child put them into words.

However, try to avoid the common pitfalls of saying things like, "Words don't hurt," or, giving advice about what to do the next time. (After all, there is no exact formula on how to react to teasing.)

Speaking directly to the friend involved, or calling his or her parents, may be useful if the friend is under 7 or 8. However, such approaches may backfire when used with older children, because they can bring even more unwanted attention to your child. But keep in mind that these are not hard and fast rules; they depend on the nature of the offense and the people involved.

Listen to your child. Stay tuned for indications that he or she doesn't fully understand the illness.

Tough Call

It's difficult to know how to help a child with diabetes deal with friends. On the one hand parents need to help a child feel like one of the crowd. Sameness gives a child more of a choice in deciding whether or not to disclose the diabetes to friends. Sameness also helps in another way. The more a child fits in with others, the more existing differences, such as having a morning snack, seem acceptable.

To cultivate sameness, your child can have school snacks that resemble everyone else's. Or, you can make snacks for the entire class on occasion.

Lunchtime testing or injections can be arranged at the nurse's office or other private area. The child can be given permission to go to the bathroom or leave the room without raising a hand or making a fuss about it. All of these accommodations help.

Remember, though, the child must want these extra measures, not the parent or the teacher. Otherwise, a youngster may feel he or she is being asked to hide the diabetes, that there is something wrong about having it.

On the other hand, parents need to help the child appreciate how he or she is different from others, but not alone. See if you can introduce your child to other people who have diabetes or other chronic illnesses. For instance, ask if your child would like to choose a pen pal from *Diabetes Forecast's* Do Write column, or put his or her own name in.

Let your youngster know that the American Diabetes Association has camps just for children with diabetes. (For information on camps, contact the American Diabetes Association affiliate in your area. You can find the phone number in the white pages.)

Branch out. Try to have your child meet people of other national, racial, or ethnic backgrounds. Such meetings reinforce the idea that diversity is common, desirable, and a normal part of the world we live in.

Peggy Finston, MD, *is a psychiatrist and the mother of two children with serious food allergies. She is the author of* Parenting Plus: Raising Children With Special Health Needs. *The book, winner of the 1992 Media Award from the President's Committee on Employment of People with Disabilities, was published by Penguin, 1992.*

21

Surviving the Preteens

by Felise Levine

Not yet a teen, no longer a child, your preteenager needs to be treated with special sensitivity. Tuesday morning your 11-year-old gets up on time, tests his or her own blood glucose, injects the appropriate amount of insulin, then eats a healthy breakfast without comment or help. Wednesday morning the same youngster needs to be called three times, complaining that testing is a nuisance, injections are painful, and breakfasts are boring. You are forced to supervise each step of your child's diabetes regimen this day while listening to a barrage of gripes. "I'm going to eat anything I feel like." "It's not fair." You may even hear the most horrible of standbys, "I hate you."

But none of this is news to you, if you're the parent of a child between 10 and 13 years of age. You're probably well aware that your son or daughter is at an in-between age when childhood activities seem infantile, but teen responsibilities are still a bit overwhelming.

Which Is Real?

Which should you respond to—the budding adult, or the insecure child? The dilemma can make even the calmest parents want to join their preteen in screaming, "I hate this." During this unpredictable period, it is important to respond to the unruly child as well as the emerging adult. This will require deft handling of a number of situations, one of the most crucial being the youngster's diabetes management.

The shift from near-total dependence to measured independence in diabetes care occurs at different times in different families. Although some experts suggest that an 11- to 13-year-old should be taking over primary responsibility for diabetes self-care, every family makes the transition at its own speed.

There is, however, one thing you probably can count on: You are likely to have a somewhat rougher time during these years than parents of children who do not have diabetes. That's because your youngster is having a rougher time, too.

The Same—But Different

Preteens with diabetes have to make all the psychological, physiological, and social adjustments that other children do. Like their friends, they must deal with hormonal changes, new nutritional needs, alterations in body image, and shifting family and peer relationships.

However, the changes occurring in these years pose unique problems for the child with diabetes. For example, the onset of puberty and the growth spurts that occur at this time of life affect insulin dosages and dietary needs, and the diabetes regimen that worked a year ago may no longer properly control blood glucose levels. So, just at the time a youngster has a psychological need for more independence, he or she has a physical requirement for more supervision in adjusting insulin dosages and diet.

Balance the need to protect your child with the necessity of letting go.

For girls, this is further complicated by the hormonal changes of the menstrual cycle. By the time a girl has her first period, her growth has started to slow down. This means her caloric requirements have decreased, and the likelihood of weight gain has increased. For her, a trip to the doctor or dietitian may mean learning that her blood glucose is too high, that she has gained weight, and that she has to watch her diet and eat less.

The problem is further complicated by the fact that a girl this age has a growing sensitivity to her body. In addition, she is now getting invited to more social events and sleepovers, most of which involve meals or snacks. All of this makes it difficult for her to stick with her diet and eat less. No doubt, the preteens are a difficult time for girls with diabetes.

Boys usually have an easier time managing their diabetes during these years because the growth spurts they experience require ever increasing amounts of calories to sustain. That's why it sometimes seems that adolescent boys with diabetes are able to eat virtually anything and not affect their blood glucose levels or become fat.

Nevertheless, the teen years present a danger to them, too, although it is delayed. Because they can get away with more, adolescent boys learn unhealthy eating habits and forget that they still have to take care of their diabetes. They may gobble down milkshakes, hamburgers, and fries and think they are fooling everybody because their blood glucose remains in the healthy range. But that's only because their adolescent bodies let them get away with a great deal. A few years later, when they reach young adulthood and their growth spurt stops, they often run into trouble because they are undisciplined about their diabetes regimen.

Growing independence is a double-edged sword in other ways, too. While all preteens have an increasing number of decisions to make, the youngster with diabetes confronts an even larger number—and with potentially more serious results.

The "tween" years are also complicated by the feelings of hopelessness and anger that often accompany a chronic illness. The preteen's desire to be on his or her own gets mixed up with the discipline of a rigorous daily regimen. And the search for identity and self-image is made more difficult because preteens with diabetes may be struggling with the sense of being different, or even "defective."

The child approaching puberty is also coming to grips with a new awareness of the possibility of diabetic complications. While you may hear, "I don't want to talk about diabetes all the time," your preteen may actually share the same worries you have about the disease and his or her future.

Facing Hypoglycemia

Like all young people, the emerging teenager with diabetes wants to be accepted, fit in, and be like everyone else. Yet diabetes defeats those wishes at every turn. Preteens with diabetes have to watch what they eat, monitor their blood sugar, keep track of their exercise levels, take insulin, and be on guard against reactions. All this seems designed to make them feel that they are different.

In addition, if the preteenager keeps tight blood glucose control, he or she risks having hypoglycemic (low blood glucose) reactions. Symptoms of an hypoglycemia, such as irritability, confusion, sweatiness, and weakness, expose the youth to possible humiliation and embarrassment in front of friends.

Even when those friends know about the diabetes, they may still not know how to distinguish between a bad mood and hypoglycemia. They may withdraw or even retaliate against a perceived "bad mood." And they may respond to the explanation, "I'm having low blood sugar. I need some candy," with, "You're just making it up so you can eat something sweet."

No wonder fear of a low blood glucose reaction can inhibit a youngster from participating in sports or overnights. In fact, the preteen may feel that he or she is actually being punished for having good control.

This may help explain why some children become lax in their diabetes care as they reach adolescence. They will do almost anything to keep from being embarrassed by a hypoglycemic reaction—even risking high blood sugars.

What About You?

As difficult as it can be for the child, diabetes in a preteen is almost as tough on you, the parent.

You want to encourage your son or daughter to become independent, but that means forcing yourself to stand by while the child you love experiments with—even jeopardizes—his or her diabetes control.

You want to ask your child's friend's parents to supervise blood glucose testing during an overnight, but your son or daughter wails that such a request is a betrayal.

You may spend sleepless hours as your child begins to stay out later. You may even find yourself worrying that your son or daughter has had low blood glucose and needs help. Yet you don't want to embarrass your child, who is trying so hard to be grown up, with a phone call to see if everything is OK.

And, when something goes wrong, you may feel like screaming, "How could you break the rules like this? How can I trust you next time?" Given a little more time, you might really want to say, "I'm so frightened for your future."

Balancing the need to protect your child with the necessity of letting go may be the most painful part of parenthood. This is especially true when your child has a chronic illness.

Here's Help

If all this sounds grim, take heart. Preteenagers are also lively, energetic, and full of new ideas as well as a growing sense of responsibility. It can be a joy to watch them open up and mature. And you can help.

For one thing, since diabetes offers a wide arena for rebellion as well as conflict, try to distinguish between diabetes and issues that are not related to diabetes.

You might say, "You can't stay out until 2 a.m. because you're too young," instead of "You cannot stay out until 2 in the morning because it would interfere with your diabetes control." The first answer is just as honest, and perhaps a little easier to take, since friends will be getting the same explanation.

Remember, too, that many of the things you worry about are simply a part of growing up for many youngsters. For instance, children this age often switch allegiances from one parent to another, and back again. That happens regardless of which parent has come down hardest on diabetes control.

When something goes awry, such as when your child's blood glucose soars to 375 mg/dl (milligrams per deciliter) following a party, hold down your panic (or your anger), and try to turn the experience into something positive. Sit down with your child and attempt to determine why his or her blood sugars climbed so high. Then see if you can come to some agreement, or develop a strategy to prevent a "next time."

It's very helpful to be sensitive to your child's signals. For instance, if your youngster has always felt comfortable going to a doctor of the opposite sex but is now making excuses to avoid appointments, it may be left to you to put two and two together.

Sensitivity to and respect for such feelings are important. So, even if you hear "You're always interfering" in the morning, and "You don't care about anything I do" in the afternoon, don't despair. Children want to move forward as much as their parents want them to.

And even on the darkest days, keep your sense of humor. After all, this process will eventually allow your youngster to go off on his or her own, leaving you proud and a little amazed at the bright, sensitive adult you've raised.

And be kind to yourself. Remember that tomorrow will bring the chance to try again.

15 Guides Through the Preteens

1. Know your child. Different children need different styles of discipline and guidance. Although a child may act grown up, his or her reasoning skills may still not be fully mature.

2. Communicate with your child. Don't assume your child knows what you are thinking, or that you know what he or she is thinking.

Discuss your rules and expectations. And when things have calmed down after a run-in, ask how your child thinks the discussion went.

If your youngster complains about how you handled a situation, try role reversal. Ask what he or she would do in your place.

3. Remember your own childhood. How would your mother or father have handled the situation? How did you feel about the things they did or said? What do you wish they would have done differently? Are you over-compensating for what your parents did or didn't do?

Get a sense of a youngster's feelings by recalling your own.

4. Don't let guilt interfere. Even though no one is to blame for a child's having diabetes, parents sometimes feel that one or the other "contributed" the culprit gene. That can create a feeling of guilt or blame, making children sense that there is a "good" and a "bad" parent.

Feeling guilty yourself, or placing blame on the other parent, undermines the parental partnership and fogs the diabetes control messages to the child.

5. Be consistent. Don't accept a rule infraction one time, then get angry at the same infraction the next time. That leaves a child confused and uncertain.

Don't make a rule you're not sure you can back up. And make sure both parents agree before you set a rule.

6. Practice parental teamwork. Don't let one parent get stuck with being the strict enforcer, while the other is the "good guy." This makes you undercut each other and leaves you unavailable to give each other support. It can produce an angry, confused preteenager who learns to divide and conquer.

It's especially important for you both to agree to reinforce each other if you are separated or divorced. Consult a professional if you can't agree on how to work as a team with your child.

7. Tolerate limited rebelliousness. Distinguish between areas where a little rebellion can be tolerated, such as resistance to the clothing choices you make, and areas where it cannot, such as resistance to injections.

Allow some negotiations on the less vital rules. It's important for a child to challenge and negotiate with authority figures once in a while.

8. Include your child in decisions. When you set rules, ask for your child's thoughts, and then express your own on the issue. "You want to stay overnight at Sarah's house, but I'm worried about you eating junk food and not testing yourself." Or, "You don't want to show me your test results every day, but I'm worried that if I don't see them, you won't test."

Give the youngster some input into solutions, but make the final decision yourself.

9. Solve rather than punish. It's unlikely that you can totally prevent your child from experimenting with diabetes care, such as sneaking food, overeating at parties, or drinking. Ultimately, these decisions will be made by the child anyway. So, instead of reacting by yelling and threatening punishment, tell your child why you are so upset.

Discuss how to be prepared for difficult situations. "What will you say if the guys tease you about refusing a drink?" or "How will you handle it when they serve the cake?" Let your child know that even if he or she makes choices that bring trouble, you will be there to help out, not to punish.

10. Shift to adult techniques. Your child is no longer at the age for, "Do it because I said so." Now it's time for negotiations, discussions, problem solving, and

choice. Ask, "What would seem fair to you?" "What would balance good diabetes control with having fun?"

11. Distinguish between diabetes and non-diabetes issues. Don't make diabetes the focal point for all decisions or disagreements. Be clear when a decision is based on other factors, such as grades, age, and the like.

12. Plan a day out from the diabetes regimen. Check with your physician. If your child is in good control, the health care team may agree to an occasional day off from some diabetes routines. This may mean no blood sugar testing, no recording of blood sugars, some additional food choices or treats, or a meal without calculations.

13. Join a parent support group. Call your local American Diabetes Association chapter and see if there is a parent support group in your area. If there isn't, consider starting one yourself. Other parents can be a valuable resource. See chapters 17 and 25.

14. Seek professional help when necessary. Some problems just can't be handled on your own. If you bump into something that isn't working out, ask your physician, diabetes educator, nurse educator, or request that your local ADA chapter recommend a psychologist, social worker, or family counselor who specializes in diabetes-related problems.

15. Forget perfection. This may be the most important advice of all. There is no such thing as perfect parents, perfect children, or perfect diabetes care. Be realistic.

Felise Levine, PhD, *who has had type 1 diabetes since age 15, is a licensed psychologist in private practice at the Center for Family and Psychological Studies in San Diego. She is the psychology consultant for the Whittier Institute for Diabetes in La Jolla. She is also chairperson of the Support Services Committee and a support group facilitator for the San Diego Chapter of the ADA California Affiliate.*

22
Stay in Touch

by Patricia D. Stenger

You've just heard the startling news. Your wonderful grandchild has been diagnosed with diabetes.

Of course, you're worried and confused, but you don't want to bother the child's mom and dad. After all, they're busy talking to doctors, making decisions, comforting their youngster, and maybe caring for other children in the family.

Where Do I Fit Now?

Still, you'd like to know what this diabetes is all about, what the future will be, and where you fit into your grandchild's life now.

Before diabetes came along, your role was clear. You were there for birthdays and holidays, perhaps special visits, and even overnights with your grandchild in your home.

If you live near your grandchild, you may also have been a babysitter and the two of

Grandparents: Want to stay in touch with your grandchild? Learn all you can about his or her diabetes.

173

you probably had outings together. Perhaps you took your grandchild to religious events, the circus, or a children's theater. It's likely you made or bought your grandchild's favorite snacks.

Now that diabetes is in the picture, how will your role change?

Now More Than Ever

Some things, of course, will stay the same. The child, and his or her parents, will need your support and love more than ever. So, keep doing all those things you've done before—have fun with your grandchild.

But there's more involved now, and you owe it to your grandchild, and to yourself, to learn all you can about diabetes. That way, you'll be able to help the child stay healthy while you help the rest of the family adjust to the change.

Up To You

Begin by checking the newspaper or calling your local American Diabetes Association chapter or state affiliate, your own doctor, or a nearby hospital. Ask about diabetes education classes. Many locations have them available at no cost.

Ask your librarian for books on diabetes, or you can call the American Diabetes Association and request a catalog of materials on the subject (1–800–DIABETES).

Consider joining, or even starting, a support group for family members of children with diabetes. You may be surprised at how many grandparents, aunts, uncles, and cousins of children with this disease live in your area.

What Will I Learn?

You'll soon understand that your grandchild has insulin-dependent (type 1) diabetes. (Generally, children and young adults have this type of diabetes. Those diagnosed after 40 have non-insulin-dependent [type 2] diabetes.)

You'll also learn that neither type of diabetes is curable, but that both are controllable. However, controlling type 1 diabetes is complex. To do that, your grandchild will be learning to balance the following elements:

* Insulin, a hormone produced in the beta cells of the pancreas, works like a key. It opens the cells and allows glucose (derived from food) to get inside. Without insulin, glucose remains in the bloodstream.

When that happens, cells do not get the energy they need to function properly and the person becomes ill.

People with insulin-dependent diabetes (and some with non-insulin-dependent diabetes) take one or more insulin injections a day. Your grandchild will need insulin for the rest of his or her life, or until researchers find a cure for this disease.

* Self-monitoring of blood glucose is an easy way to tell how much glucose is in the bloodstream.

Your grandchild will be monitoring his or her blood glucose several times a day, every day. That means the child (or an adult) will prick the child's finger, obtain a drop of blood, and use it with a meter the size of a pocket calculator to get a reading.

Before self-monitoring of blood glucose was developed, people with diabetes had to test their urine to find out if their diabetes was in control. Or, they went to the doctor to have their blood glucose tested, but they only did that every few months. What's more, by the time the result came back from the laboratory a few days later, the person's blood glucose levels had altered so much that the results were almost irrelevant.

Grandparent in Charge

For Yourself

* Learn all you can about insulin-dependent (type 1) diabetes. Read books and magazines; attend classes; ask questions; perhaps join or start a family support group.
* Rid yourself of any guilt feelings you may have if there is diabetes in your family. No one really knows why one person gets the disease and not another.
* Don't feel anger at your son or daughter's spouse, if diabetes is on that side of the family.
* Keep diabetes equipment, as well as appropriate food, available in your home. That will make it easier for your grandchild to visit you.
* Post the phone number and the directions to the nearest hospital emergency room near your phone. Also post the child's doctor's phone number.
* Be firm with your grandchild when firmness is necessary to keep him or her in good diabetes control.
* Maintain the diabetes regimen. Don't sneak food to the child, or say things like, "It's OK just this once."

For Your Family

* Praise the parents and siblings, as well as the child, for handling diabetes so well.
* Once you are educated about diabetes, offer to babysit for an evening or a weekend.
* Don't be pushy. If you receive a turndown, accept it. You might offer an alternative date or simply say, "I'm here when you need me."
* Make suggestions about the child's care to the parents when you are alone with them. Don't criticize the parents in front of the child.

* Ask the parents—in private—if it's OK to invite your grandchild for a visit on a given date. Wait until you have the parents' OK before asking the child.
* If the parents turn down your invitation, don't make them "the bad guys" by letting the child know about the turndown.
* Nobody agrees with others all the time. If you have a problem with a parental decision, don't let your anger fester and grow. Talk about it, but pick a time when no one is angry or harried.
* Remember that the parents are in charge, even if they are young and inexperienced. While your love goes directly to the child, your plans should go through the parents.

Now self-monitoring of blood glucose can let you know the level of glucose in the blood any time, day or night. That not only helps the doctor choose the appropriate type of insulin to be used (short, intermediate, or long-lasting) and the amount of each dose, but it also provides information about blood glucose levels during special circumstances, such as when the child participates in athletics, or attends a party.

* A healthy meal plan, as you probably know, is a mainstay of diabetes management. Eating appropriately will go a long way toward keeping your grandchild healthy.

Mom and Dad and the child with diabetes may visit a registered dietitian (RD) who will set up a food plan, or learn about nutrition from the doctor or a certified diabetes educator (CDE). If possible, go along on this visit, or talk to a registered dietitian yourself.

In any case, don't despair. Your grandchild's food plan can certainly contain items he or she enjoys. What's more, it's easy to make appropriate choices with the new

Nutrition Facts and Ingredient labels and the wide selection of foods in today's market.

Don't be overly worried about sugar either. It's no longer a forbidden food for people with diabetes. Again, talk to health professionals, read, and educate yourself on nutrition. You'll find that a healthy diet for someone with diabetes is virtually the same as a healthy diet for everyone.

* Exercise will also be a pillar of your grandchild's diabetes care. That's because exercise not only keeps the body healthy, but also plays a part in how the body uses insulin.

What Do I Need To Know?

Once you understand the basics of good diabetes control, you'll learn a few other vital pieces of information.

The most important is how to recognize an insulin reaction—low blood glucose—and what to do about it. This is a serious event that requires immediate action. It would not be wise for you to care for your grandchild on your own until you understand insulin reactions.

Although our bodies need insulin, and people with diabetes inject insulin, the body can have too much of a good thing. Excessive insulin in the bloodstream can cause your grandchild's blood glucose (also called blood sugar) to plummet.

When that happens, the person with diabetes needs food that turns to glucose quickly. In other words, he or she needs some form of sugar.

That might be orange juice, cake decorating gel, nondiet soda, or a form of glucose you can purchase. If the situation is serious, you may need to inject glucagon, or get the child to an emergency room quickly.

You'll learn to understand, recognize, and treat insulin reactions in your diabetes classes.

Timing, Discipline

Timing is also an important element in diabetes control. The body must have some insulin available before food is consumed.

Add the fact that different types of insulins are active in the body for varying time periods, and you'll see why it's important for your grandchild to take insulin and to eat and snack at specific times.

Discipline comes into play too. Although grandparents are wonderfully famous for bending rules where a grandchild is concerned, there are times when you have to be firm.

It will be more helpful and loving for you to say, "Sorry, that isn't the best snack," than for you to let the child eat something inappropriate.

However, rest assured that you and your grandchild can still go to restaurants, eat, cook, and bake together—as long as you are "up" on what foods and quantities are appropriate for your grandchild. They're probably the same ones that are appropriate for you.

Insider

Once you learn about diabetes, you'll feel like an insider. You won't be confused when your son or daughter says, "Stacy's sugar is up a bit today," or "It's time for Bob's glucose check."

You'll be able to help with insulin injections and blood glucose checks, too, if you wish. And your family will know they can rely on your advice, or ask you to be a sounding board when a decision has to be made.

You can even answer questions and help educate your grandchild about diabetes. As an adult, your picture of the disease will probably be clearer than his or hers.

Also, if you feel any guilt because there is diabetes in your family, education will show you what a complex disease diabetes is. Even with years of research, scientists are not entirely sure how or why it develops in one person and not in another. And no one is responsible for his or her genes.

After you've learned about diabetes, let your family know that you have attended classes and read up on the subject. Express your self-confidence. Assure everyone that you can now give your grandchild appropriate physical as well as emotional care.

Once you are knowledgeable about diabetes care, you can step in and give Mom and Dad a well-earned day, night, or weekend off.

You can help reassure the other children, too. Let them know their brother or sister will be fine. That they cannot "catch" diabetes, and that they are still very much loved, even if their newly diagnosed brother or sister is getting all the attention just now.

Education will allow you to provide the shoulder the rest of the family cries on during this crisis. It will enable you to be a source of strength and support, a role supremely suited to grandparents.

Knowing about diabetes will allay other concerns, too. You'll see that diabetes care today is a far cry from what it was only a few years ago. Self-monitoring of blood glucose, for example, is a fairly recent advancement in diabetes management.

A Few Words

Diabetes Mellitus—A disease that occurs when the body is unable to process sugar properly.

There are two main types of diabetes. In insulin-dependent (type 1) diabetes, the pancreas makes virtually no insulin. This type of diabetes usually appears suddenly in children and young adults and requires insulin injections.

In non-insulin-dependent (type 2) diabetes, the pancreas either makes an inadequate amount of insulin, or the body cannot use insulin properly. This type can develop slowly and usually occurs in people after age 40. It's generally treated by medication and diet. Approximately 90 percent of the people who have diabetes have type 2.

Glucose—A simple form of sugar. The body changes most of the food we eat into glucose, and glucose then fuels the body's cells.

Glucagon—A hormone produced by the alpha cells of the pancreas. It raises the level of glucose in the blood. A person who is unconscious because of a serious insulin reaction requires an injection of glucagon.

Insulin—A hormone produced by the beta cells of a healthy pancreas. Insulin functions as a kind of key to open the body's cells. Once they are open, glucose can enter the cells and give them energy.

Insulin Reaction—An event that can come about when there is low blood sugar in the body. Low blood sugar is generally caused by excessive insulin or not enough carbohydrate-containing food.

An insulin reaction must be treated with some form of sugar immediately. Symptoms include sweating, shakiness, dizziness, and confusion.

Ketones—Acids formed by the body when it burns fat instead of glucose for energy. Ketones in the body are a warning that the diabetes is not well controlled.

You will also realize that your grandchild can eat tasty foods, join an athletic team, sleep at friends' homes, take trips, plan for the future, and enjoy all the fun of growing up that other kids do.

And you'll surely be pleased at the invaluable gift you gave yourself, your family, and your grandchild, when you took the trouble to educate yourself about diabetes.

"I Love You, Grandma and Grandpa"

As a grandparent, you play an important role in your grandchild's life. You bring the child a sense of the past, of continuity, of belonging to a larger group. You open the child's eyes to other stages of life and to other lifestyles.

Something will be missing if you are not involved in some way in your grandchild's life, whatever your "grandparenting" style.

You may love to roll on the floor with the kids, or you may be a bit more formal. You may want to be in on all the details of your grandchild's life, or deal mainly with special occasions. But even if you live far away, it's a good idea to stay in touch. Exchange tapes of yourself with your grandchild's family. Remember birthdays, holidays, graduations, and other special days. Drop a note for no reason at all. Children love mail addressed to them. Pick up the phone and call once in awhile, if you can.

No matter how you handle it, you, grandmother and grandfather, bring a kind of love to your grandchild that no one else can duplicate.

Patricia D. Stenger, RN, CDE, *past Senior Vice President of the American Diabetes Association, is a diabetes educator at the Eastern Maine Medical Center in Bangor. She is also director of Camp Kee-to-Kin, a camp for families that have a child with diabetes, and Camp Grand, a camp for grandparents and their grandchildren with diabetes.*

23

Quitting the Self-Blame Game

by Peggy Finston

I f you feel guilty about your child's diabetes, check out this second opinion.

Many men and women become fathers and
mothers believing they will be perfect parents. They expect to protect, nurture, and
guide their child into adulthood in the best
mental and physical health possible. But if
that child is diagnosed with insulin-dependent (type 1) diabetes, their naive and comforting fantasy can wash away with the first
insulin injection. Crushed and saddened, the
confused parent's first question is often,
"What did I do wrong?"

A Common Denominator: Guilt

Psychiatrists find that when any disability or
chronic illness afflicts a child, it is common

for parents to blame themselves. And because diabetes has a genetic component, it's easy for a parent to express that blame by deciding that he or she is "guilty" of passing on a defective gene. Or, a parent may take the opposite approach, and search his or her family tree to prove that the "bad genes" did not originate there.

Either way, it's the same game that's being played: Pin the blame on the parent.

If this were the only guilt that parents experience, they might be able to find a way to handle it.

But parents of children with diabetes are vulnerable to feeling guilty about a host of things. They sometimes blame themselves for not seeing the problem sooner, or for discounting signs of the illness, such as increased thirst or unexplained weight loss, as if not recognizing these signs means they were negligent, or that such recognition could have altered the diagnosis.

Parents may also blame themselves for not being able to protect their child from both the physical pain of treatments and tests and the emotional pain of "being different."

Mothers, in particular, are all too ready to indict themselves when they have a child with special needs. Some flail themselves almost daily with the question, "Am I doing the best I can for this child?" Self-accusation can plague their lives.

Parents who have several children often add another measure of guilt by giving extra time to the child with diabetes, then feeling they are neglecting their other children.

What these parents don't do is give themselves a break for the difficulties they face, the decisions they must make that other parents aren't even aware of. After all, these parents have to figure out how to give their child the best diabetes care possible while making sure the daily routine of testing, injecting, exercising, and careful eating doesn't restrict other aspects of their youngster's daily life.

They also have to weigh the substantial sums of money they spend for a child with special needs against the requirements of the rest of the family.

Those are tall orders for any parent, and there are no right and wrong ways to handle them. Yet some mothers and fathers have such a sense of guilt, such a negative view of themselves, that they can't believe that their decisions are likely to be as wise as anyone else's.

Guilt Has Many Teachers

The surprise is that, although the guilt that parents feel is complex, it generally has little to do with the reality of the child's condition or their own actions. Parental guilt generally springs not from things parents did or did not do, but from deeper, less rational sources.

Guilt has many teachers.

One of the strongest is society's sexual stereotypes of men and women. Despite recent attempts to redefine parental roles, many women still see themselves as total nurturers; many fathers still feel they have to be perfect protectors. These ingrained stereotypes impose impossible standards on any parent. To one raising a child with a chronic illness, they can be devastating.

Or, some parents may misunderstand religious teachings and feel that they are being punished through their child's illness. Those who come from families that emphasize achievement and success may see their child's illness as their personal failure.

An even more irrational source of guilt arises from a latent, childlike view of the world that sees the self as all-powerful. (This is the view that can make a child feel responsible for a tornado because he or she wanted someone's picnic spoiled.)

Many crises—from being the victim of a crime to being the parent of a youngster with a chronic illness—bring adults back to that same sense of being responsible for everything. They then grill themselves with the thought, "If only I had done it this way, things would be different."

The Harm That Guilt Brings

Although guilt is often enmeshed in positive, loving feelings, it can do real harm to the entire family.

Once a parent accepts guilt, it can open the door to a continuous string of negative judgments on virtually every decision he or she makes. This parent may decide that it was a mistake to leave a child with a sitter, permit a child to join an athletic team, or even allow a son or daughter to go to school without a sweater.

Parents who fall prey to feelings of guilt may also decide they are incompetent and unworthy to be parents. But the problem doesn't end there. The child usually senses their unhappiness and may, in turn, feel responsible for it, perhaps thinking, "If I didn't have diabetes, everything would be OK."

Clearly, parents need to manage their sense of guilt, if not for their own sakes, then for that of their children.

Dealing With Guilt

There are things people can do to help allay their sense of guilt, or at least help them learn to live with it.

One time-tested method for ridding oneself of emotional demons is to confess them to someone else.

Whether this confession takes place with a member of the clergy, a mental health professional, mentor, good friend, or within a support group, it can be very beneficial. But the talk needs to be ongoing. It takes time to change the way we perceive the world.

Another way to deal with guilt is to accept it and move past it. Things are the way they are; guilt won't change them. One mother of a child with diabetes said to me, "I finally came to a place where I realized there was nothing I could do. No matter how I blamed myself, my daughter was going to live with diabetes, and I had to live with that fact."

A similar approach suggests putting guilt in its place. Acknowledge the feeling, but don't berate yourself every minute. Another mother of a child with this illness told me, "I get fed up every so often, and then I feel guilty. But I see my guilt as an involuntary reflex, and I know that feeling guilty doesn't mean that I don't care about my child."

Feelings, even intense feelings, do not necessarily reflect reality.

The Big Picture

Whether a parent has strong religious convictions or not, nurturing some kind of "big picture" concept of the world can go a long way toward relieving guilt. Such a concept can lessen one's sense of being all-powerful. It helps a parent acknowledge that many events are simply beyond his or her control.

One way to realize this is to learn about the disease itself. Once a parent grasps the objective reality of diabetes, he or she can begin to understand that nobody is to blame.

Knowledge can also prepare parents for some down times. The course of diabetes, as with any chronic illness, does not always run smoothly. If the child has an insulin reaction, or an undesirable blood glucose reading, parents should know that insulin reactions happen and that blood glucose readings go high or low for a variety of reasons, some of them not even clearly understood.

It's important that parents not let these problems generate even more guilt within themselves. The more parents know about the disease, the greater will be their ability to roll with the punches, and even come up with possible solutions.

"I Love You, Mommy and Daddy"

Finally, parents who feel guilty or incompetent should try to look at themselves in a new way. They should try to see that it is their passionate attachment to their children that enables their son or daughter to survive crises and to prosper. It is their love that feeds their child's self-esteem.

All parents should take time to notice what they are doing right for their family. They should remember how they have brought their children through difficult days and teary nights, provided medical care, needed supplies, and healthy foods. They comfort and care for this child, share the sadness and join in the laughter, all significant parts of being a good parent.

And when the youngster has a success—starts school, goes to camp, makes the team—parents should recognize the occasions. They can mark the dates on their own calendars, acknowledge their help in forging these victories, relish them, and give themselves a great big pat on the back.

Peggy Finston, MD, *is a mother of two children with food allergies and the author of* Parenting Plus: Raising Children With Special Health Needs, *the 1991 winner of the President's Committee on Employment of People with Disabilities' media award.*

24

Games Couples Play

These games don't depend on a roll of the dice or a hand of cards. They're not the well-known diversions of Monopoly, Scrabble, or Bridge, but for many couples they are familiar pastimes. In fact, psychological games are anything but trivial pursuits.

by Matti K. Gershenfeld

The scene is the dining room table. Jane and Howard are having their evening meal, and, as usual, it's their first chance to talk about the day's events.

JANE: What did the doctor say when you went there today? How are you?

HOWARD: I don't remember what he said. You know, he mumbles.

JANE: Well, think about it. What did he say?

HOWARD: I don't remember, I told you. I don't remember a thing he said.

JANE: Well, are you supposed to increase your insulin? What did he say about your weight? Have you gained weight?

HOWARD: Will you stop bugging me! I don't remember! I told you!

The next morning, Jane calls the doctor. She writes down the information about Howard's weight and insulin and the doctor's comments. That night, Howard comes home, sees the note, and screams, "You're always trying to control me! You're always meddling, telling me what to do. You have to control everything!" Jane starts to cry. "This always happens," she says. "Every time you go to the doctor, we have a fight."

On the surface, the issues seem simple: Howard doesn't want Jane interfering in his medical affairs; Jane wants to be a supportive partner who helps Howard stay in good health. Both people seem reasonable, and yet Howard's trips to the doctor always end in a fight. Why? Why doesn't Howard—a successful, intelligent executive—simply ask the doctor for the information he needs? Why does Jane continue to call the doctor when she knows that she'll be accused of meddling?

Howard and Jane are locked into this struggle because they are playing out a psychological game called "I'm Really A Baby." Like many couples, they are substituting a familiar pattern of behavior for a direct discussion about a diabetes-related problem.

Having diabetes is often frightening—it can cause people to feel vulnerable and insecure. Sometimes, living with diabetes can erode an individual's self-esteem. Previously secure, loving partners can find themselves questioning whether they are still attractive to their mate. Rather than facing their fears and insecurities, couples often resort to psychological games that let them feel—at least momentarily—in control.

All couples play psychological games at one time or another. Games provide a familiar structure for getting a predictable response. Often games give one of the players a short term feeling of satisfaction. (I won! She's wrong and I'm right!) Games, when they prove a long-held belief (diabetes makes me unlovable), can make life seem predictable and safe.

While some game playing in relationships is inevitable, substituting psychological games for honest discussions can spell trouble. Usually games leave both partners feeling angry or hurt. Though someone has "won," it is usually at the expense of closeness and intimacy. Eventually, games create barriers to sharing and direct conversations. The result is often increasing distance between partners.

How can we understand Howard and Jane's game? If they could talk to each other honestly, it would become clear that Howard is terrified of having diabetes. When he thinks about the future, he imagines only bleak possibilities. Although he appears to be a strong, competent, successful adult, inside he feels frightened and alone. His fear makes it difficult to concentrate on the doctor's comments. At some level, he wants Jane to help and take care of him. He knows she loves him and wants to be helpful. Yet, his self-image doesn't allow him to ask for help; after all, he is supposed to take care of her. It makes him feel like a baby to ask Jane, "Come to the doctor with me—I'm scared," or "Remind me to write out everything so that I will retain it." He prefers to go through this game of feeling angry that Jane "nags him" about what the doctor said. He wants her to get the information for him, but somehow cannot acknowledge that it is helpful. Instead, he yells at her for controlling him and meddling. Jane ends up with her usual feeling— "No matter what I do, it's wrong."

End Game

The good news is that games can be stopped. The first step in ending a game is recognizing that you are a player. Often, this isn't as simple as it sounds. People do not realize they are playing games; they think they are acting naturally. For example, if Jane accused Howard of playing a game, he would innocently respond, "I don't know what you're talking about."

For some people, games are the main way of interacting with others. These individuals may need professional help to change. Working with a skilled therapist (especially a therapist trained in Transactional Analysis) may help them understand how and why they play games and learn alternative, more satisfying and successful, ways of developing intimacy with others.

Other people who resort to game playing only occasionally may be able to help themselves.

Let's look at some common games couples play around diabetes, beginning with "I'm Only Trying To Help."

Karen has diabetes. She has asked her husband, John, to come with her for her regular doctor's visits. His going is a demonstration of his caring. But here's how a typical visit goes:

DOCTOR: How are you? How's your blood sugar running?

KAREN: About 200–250.

JOHN: She's lying. Last Saturday, it was up to 500.

KAREN: (Ignoring John) I exercise regularly. I walk everyday.

JOHN: She never walks on weekends.

KAREN: (Glares at John) I've been feeling fine. I haven't had any "weak" times.

JOHN: Last Saturday, this weakness came over her, and she couldn't get out of bed.

KAREN: (Very angry) Will you stop interrupting me!

JOHN: I'm only trying to help.

As they leave the doctor's office, John says angrily, "We have this fight every time we come to the doctor's. You don't appreciate all I do for you!"

What is this game about? In the doctor's office, Karen paints a picture of herself as being a model patient in good control. But while she's trying to show the doctor how good she's been, John notes every time she's lying.

If Karen wants to tell the story her way, why does she bring John? Or, why doesn't she say, "I'm going to see the doctor; you sit outside in the waiting room." One possible explanation for Karen's behavior is that at some level, she wants the doctor to know the truth. But she also wants the doctor to think well of her, and she finds it difficult to say that she cheated.

Why does John play the game? Perhaps acting out this pattern meets a need John has to feel as if he's honest; he is straightening his wife out; he is a good person willing to incur her wrath. (He collects purity points.) He also may play the game because he knows the payoff (the doctor hearing the truth) is good for her.

How can Karen and John stop this game? First, they could notice that a pattern is occurring every time they go to the doctor. Karen might understand that she can answer the doctor's questions truthfully and the doctor will accept her even if she's not perfect. And, more important, she can realize that her relationship with John will improve if she doesn't set him up in the bad guy role.

Second, John could choose not to let Karen put him in the position of correcting her in front of the doctor. Instead, he could tell Karen directly, "I don't like correcting you and calling you a liar. I won't come with you anymore if that's how you set me up." Third, Karen and John together can recognize the game they've been playing and create a way to stop. For example, John might continue to go with Karen, but when she replies to a question with a half-truth, he might pull on his earlobe as a signal to her that she isn't telling the whole story. She might then modify her reply, "My blood sugar was mostly 200–250, but last week there were three days when it was 500." They could even laugh at this new system they've invented, building a new level of closeness in their relationship. Instead of playing out a hurtful game, John can now help Karen with her desire to be perfect in the doctor's eyes.

We Never Have Fun

Thursday afternoon, Helen made arrangements with the Joneses to get together at a new restaurant on Friday night for dinner. David has just come home from work, and she's explained the Friday night plans.

DAVID: So...we're going to that new Restaurant Tres Cher? Well, it's expensive, but it'll be worth it. The French food there is supposed to be out of this world.

HELEN: Hmm. Just remember your diabetes. You've got to be careful about those sauces. You just can't eat all those rich sauces.

DAVID: I know. I know. Don't worry.

HELEN: And when they bring the dessert cart with all those pastries, you're going to have to say, "No." Even if it's included with dinner...

DAVID: Okay, okay!

HELEN: And remember you can't get carried away with the wine...

DAVID: I won't!

HELEN: And don't forget...

DAVID: (Angry) Just forget it! Call up and cancel. I won't have a good time. You're impossible.

And, so they stay home. He's angry at her for ruining the evening. She's angry at him because life is so boring; she feels like they never go out any more. Both David and Helen are frustrated by this situation. It doesn't make sense. David wants to go out and try this new restaurant; he enjoys socializing with the Joneses. Helen wants to go out, too.

Why are they fighting? In any game, the players may have a number of reasons for playing. One possible explanation for Helen and David's game might be something common to many couples—mind reading.

Helen may have followed the Joneses' suggestion to eat at the Restaurant Tres Cher. She couldn't say that she thought it was too expensive. She also couldn't ask her husband if they could afford it. When she told him that she had made dinner plans, he said two things: He would like to go, and it was expensive. For some reason, Helen felt a need to make him look good and make herself feel bad (like a martyr). She knows he gets annoyed when she mothers him and harps on what he can and can't eat. In response to David's comments about the cost of the dinner, she finds herself saying, "Don't eat this and don't eat that." At some level, she knows that if she keeps it up long enough, he'll get angry and cancel the evening. While she'll feel badly, she'll also feel relieved that they didn't have to spend all that money. Now, he won't get angry at her later for making plans to go out for a dinner that they couldn't afford.

It's an expensive way to save a few dollars. Both Helen and David end the game feeling angry, hurt, and depressed. They could avoid this game by talking more directly to each other.

For example, when the Joneses suggested the Restaurant Tres Cher, Helen could have said, "I would love to see you, but let's pick a less expensive spot." Or, when David learned of the plans, he could have said,

"I'd really like to see the Joneses, but I don't think our budget can stand the Tres Cher. Why don't you call them and see if we can go to a less expensive place. Or, you could invite them here for the evening."

Another way to stop the game would be for Helen to present the plan to her husband and say, "I know it's expensive, but do you think we could afford it this one time?" Then, David can say, "Yes" or "No." In this way they're making plans by asking each other, not by mind reading. Games can be stopped by either partner in a number of ways.

Undercover Games

While couples want intimacy and closeness, they often sabotage themselves in sexual games. Because diabetes can induce sexual dysfunction, problems should first be checked out with a physician (urologist) to determine whether the cause is physiological or psychological. Sometimes decreased emotional satisfaction from sexual activity and lack of sexual desire are more related to psychological than physiological factors.

A chronic illness such as diabetes can sometimes result in a person feeling undesirable or insecure. Rather than recognizing these very real fears, couples often find it easier to construct games for protection against embarrassment or disappointment, or to enact a self-fulfilling prophecy. (No one could want me if I have diabetes.) Here are two examples of sexual games that couples can play around diabetes.

Diabetes Means No Sex Life

Last summer Jim turned 45 years old. He's an avid tennis player and prides himself on being physically fit. He and his wife usually make love once a week. He started to feel tired all the time and extremely thirsty. He went to the doctor and discovered that he had diabetes.

A month later, his behavior toward his wife changed substantially. He no longer initiated any interest in lovemaking. His wife pretended not to notice and said nothing.

Neither Jim nor his wife made any mention of the cessation in their lovemaking. Instead, they both talked about how busy they were or how tired they felt. He said how hard work was. By the time he read the paper at night, he was ready to go to bed. She said she was wrapped up in several projects and felt pressured at work. It went on for six months. No fighting, no arguments, no lovemaking of any kind. Then suddenly one day, Jim's wife blurted out, "Your mid-life crisis has turned you into an old man—there's no more sex!" Jim was hurt.

Why would they both ignore the situation for so long? Why would his wife try to blame the distance in their relationship on a mid-life crisis? What about Jim's feelings? Not only is he trying to deal with having diabetes, but increasingly he's feeling strained around his wife.

While there could be a number of reasons for this couple's behavior, one possible explanation has to do with Jim's reaction to the diagnosis of diabetes. When Jim was diagnosed, he was in shock and depressed. He considered himself something of a jock and prided himself on staying fit. Now, he wasn't sure how diabetes would affect his love of sports. He had also heard stories that diabetes frequently results in impotence. Shortly after his diagnosis, he was making love with his wife and had difficulty maintaining an erection. This can be a problem for middle-aged men whether or not they have diabetes. However, in his depressed state, Jim felt his worst fears were coming true. With this difficulty in lovemaking, he concluded, on a subconscious level, that he would never again be a good lover and (again subconsciously) decided not to risk the humiliation of being impotent. By pretending he wasn't interested in sex, he could protect himself from potential embarrassment. Because he didn't recognize his fear, he could not very well discuss it with his wife.

At the same time, Jim's wife had also heard that diabetes sometimes resulted in impotence. She didn't want to pressure Jim, so she pretended not to notice his lack of interest in lovemaking. Month after month they grew more and more distant, Jim feeling like a failure and his wife feeling burdened with a husband who had diabetes. Finally, enraged and frustrated, she lashed out at Jim for being an "old man" and having a "mid-life crisis."

Instead of playing a game around this problem, Jim and his wife could have done several things. They might have talked to each other and decided to try again. If the psychological impotence continued, they might have decided to see a therapist. Jim and his wife could have continued a close, loving relationship with kissing, hugging, and physical closeness. (Note: In some couples where diabetes is newly diagnosed and there is impotence, the situation is cured when the patient becomes stabilized on a diet and there is metabolic control.)

I'll Go Through the Motions

Susan, 34, has had diabetes since she was 8. Lately, she's just been going through the motions of accepting her husband's initiation of sexual advances in bed. She didn't turn him down, but she wasn't responsive either. In the evenings, they often got into fights. They had what sounded like a classic argument:

SHE: You always want to have sex.

HE: Well, you never want to.

SHE: I never turn you down, do I?

HE: It's like making love to a stone.

SHE: Well, you just don't turn me on. You're not much of a lover.

Eventually, he says, "What's the use," and slams out of the house. She feels badly and worries that it's only a matter of time before he leaves her. She wants to be close to him, but just doesn't feel sexually responsive. She often worries, "I have diabetes. I'm getting sicker. More things are going to go wrong with me. Who could possibly want me?"

Why is this couple locked into this game? It's not at all unusual that low self-esteem will produce a lack of arousal and an inability to be responsive in lovemaking. Some research suggests that there is little or no connection between a woman's ability to have an orgasm and diabetic neuropathy (nerve damage). It is rather more likely that Susan's lack of desire stems from psychological sources. Perhaps her main sense of herself is as a diabetic. By seeing herself as undesirable, she may bring about many kinds of sexual dysfunction, from lack of arousal to being non-orgasmic to complaining of pain in intercourse. As with Jim in the previous example, she does this subconsciously in an attempt to avoid future relations that she believes will lead to rejection.

Basically, she is acting out a self-fulfilling prophecy: If she is diabetic, no one could love her. The payoff of this game is that she makes her prophecy come true.

Often people with diabetes who play this type of sexual game could stop the game by talking to their partners and expressing their fears that having diabetes is making them undesirable and unlovable. They could also tell their partners they need more hugging and "I love you's" to reassure them that having diabetes does not make them a pariah.

It's Your Move

Many of the games couples play can be stopped. Most couples want intimacy and companionship from their relationship. Games played around diabetes can drive an invisible wedge between partners and become an impenetrable barrier to communication. Sometimes, coping with diabetes can lead to reduced self-esteem, depression, and fears about illness. Often these psychological pressures can affect the sexual realm of a couple's relationship and lead to more game playing.

On the other hand, adjusting to and accepting diabetes can lead to a closer bond; as couples grow together, they can help each other through both good times and bad. Learning to live with a major illness can clarify for each partner just how important the relationship is and how much each person needs the other. For some couples, this brings a new understanding that nurturing each other and being close is what each wants from the relationship. Couples can stop playing destructive games around diabetes and instead work toward direct interactions that give them pleasure, satisfaction, and mutual support.

Block That Pass

Learning how to block a game is not always simple. Some games develop over the years and even have their beginnings in childhood patterns. The needs and feelings which games develop around are often deep-seated and, therefore, hard to recognize and honestly interpret.

But ending a game being played around an aspect of diabetes is not so difficult. It can be stopped if the couple decides they'd prefer a better life with more direct interaction.

Here are some steps to bring game playing to a halt:

1. Think about arguments with your partner. Do they usually take place around specific events such as a doctor's visit, a party, or a meal in a restaurant? Do you find yourself arguing about the same things, with no real resolution? These repetitive patterns are a sign that a game is being played.

2. When you've identified the circumstances of the game, try to identify the payoff you or your partner gets from it. Although both of you may feel hurt and angry after a game, each of you "gets" something from playing it. In "I'm Really A Baby," for example, when Jane "rescues" Howard, she feels powerful. However, the real payoff of this game is Howard's. He gets the medical information he needs and also gets to play that he doesn't need Jane's help.

3. Imagine why the person who gets the main payoff needs to play the game. For example, Howard needs information from his doctor. However, fear of diabetes is keeping him from talking directly with the doctor. If Howard understood his fears, he would not need the game. Sometimes uncovering the feeling or need underlying a game can start an open discussion with your partner. It's hard to say, "I'm afraid of what the doctor might tell me," but it's harder still to keep playing the game.

4. Another step is to refuse to participate. Think about how the game escalates. How does the person who needs the payoff get things started? Howard appears indifferent about his health so that Jane will take responsibility for calling the doctor. Jane buys into the game by making the call. She could stop the game by simply not calling the doctor. Or, she could tell Howard directly, "I'm not going to let you set me up like this. I'll call the doctor if you'd like, but not if you continue to get angry with me."

5. If you're still in a rut, brainstorm with your partner about alternatives to the same old game. Once you recognize a game's underway, you can signal your partner with a nonverbal cue, like the couple in "I'm Only Trying to Help." You can put on the brakes by refusing to give the expected response. Or, you can defuse the situation by catching yourselves in the game, and laughing together at the familiar pattern. Remember, games can be stopped at any time, by either player.

Matti Gershenfeld, EdD, DHL, *would like to acknowledge the assistance of David Capuzzi, MD, PhD, in verifying the medical accuracy of this article. Dr. Gershenfeld is a Fellow of the American Association of Marriage and Family Therapy, an Adjunct Professor in the graduate school at Temple University, and member of the graduate faculty at Pennsylvania State University. In addition, she is president of the Couples Learning Center and has done extensive work with couples. Dr. Gershenfeld also has diabetes and is a board member of the Philadelphia ADA Affliate. She tries not to play psychological games with her husband.*

25
Giving Support

What is your role when someone you love has diabetes?

by Bonnie Murray

Most articles about diabetes are meant for the person with the disease. Not this one.

This is written for those who live, work, or play with someone else who has diabetes—either insulin-dependent (type 1) or non-insulin dependent (type 2).

Living with someone who has a chronic illness is difficult at times. If you have a family member with diabetes, you might want to look at how other people have handled the same kind of situation.

As a nurse, I've learned many coping skills from my patients, their spouses and families, as well as from psychologists and support groups. As the wife of a man with insulin-dependent (type 1) diabetes, I have learned other skills "the hard way."

Here is some of the information I have gathered.

First, Education

Although you are not the person who has been diagnosed with diabetes, it's a good idea for you to become informed about the disease and its treatment. That will not only help you cope, it will reassure the family member that you care enough to take an interest, to understand what he or she is going through.

Use books, magazines, pamphlets, libraries, support groups, and medical professionals as resources. Attend diabetes education classes, either with the person who has diabetes, or on your own. Try going along to some of the doctor's appointments, and keep a running list of questions or topics you wish to discuss with the doctor, nurse, or diabetes educator. Whenever possible, ask questions as they arise.

Stay on top of recent developments. Diabetes treatment has been changing dramatically in the past years. Make sure your information is up-to-date.

Caretaker or Support Person?

Sometimes it's hard to draw the line between being supportive and being the caretaker for someone you love. Yet, they are not the same.

Although there are times when you have to intervene physically in someone's diabetes care, it's usually best to steer clear of giving direct help. That's because it's important to foster the greatest possible level of independence in someone with diabetes, whether adult or child. Such independence increases feelings of self-worth.

It also helps prevent family members or friends from assuming too much of the caretaker role.

Also, when you are not enmeshed in the daily diabetes care, you're in a better position to see how well it's working.

Whenever possible, allow the person with diabetes to do his or her own blood glucose testing and insulin injecting. Let your family member make his or her own food choices.

Although not everyone is capable of the same degree of self-care, it's surprising what a little creative thinking can do when there's a problem. For instance, most people with diabetes who are vision-impaired can still self-inject if someone else prefills the syringe.

Keep in mind that allowing someone to be independent does not mean you don't care. It means, rather, that you do.

Sometimes people think they are being kind when they encourage a lax attitude in diabetes care. Saying "Go ahead, eat it, it won't hurt" is not a kindness. The real love lies in helping someone follow a self-care plan.

The daughter of a patient of mine kept bringing her father donuts, because she couldn't stand to see him deprived of something he loved. The result was that his glucose was out of control and he developed severe complications. "Depriving" him would have been an act of love.

Sometimes you can show your support simply by giving a sympathetic ear to someone who is feeling a little down, having trouble following a meal plan or with taking daily injections.

People need to talk. They need to feel someone cares about what they are going through. That's as true of someone on tight control who rarely has high blood sugars as it is of someone who is much more lax. Those on tight control feel guilty if they cheat even a little. They need someone to tell them that, realistically, it's impossible to achieve perfect control.

Those who have frequent high blood sugars and know they are not making healthy food choices certainly don't feel good about themselves. They may find it helpful to talk it out.

If you live with someone who makes excuses about his or her eating habits to you, that's your signal to ask that person to talk. Ask the family member how he or she feels about diabetes, meal plans, goals, and expectations.

Peace Of Mind

When someone you love has a chronic illness, there is no way you can avoid being concerned.

One way to help your peace of mind, however, is to make sure that the person wears an up-to-date medical identification bracelet, especially if he or she is insulin-dependent.

You'll also feel better if you know the family member will be taken care of at work or school. That's why it's good to make sure people outside the home know the symptoms of hypoglycemia (low blood sugar) and understand what to do if it occurs. If a young person is involved, it's wise to make sure school personnel can recognize low blood sugar problems and give appropriate care.

If your family member or friend with diabetes resists the idea of letting others know, talk about it. Ask about his or her fears or reservations, and try to answer each of them.

Besides the obvious health benefits to the person with diabetes, it's reassuring for you to know that someone you love will get the necessary care in an emergency, even if you are not there to give it.

What About Your Life?

Living with someone who has diabetes, either insulin-dependent or non-insulin-dependent, can impose some restrictions on your own lifestyle.

You can decide that these restrictions make you a victim, asking "Why me?" Or, you can look at them as an opportunity to better your own health habits. Think of your attention to your own health care as a gift that these special circumstances have brought you. Taking good care of yourself may help increase the quality—maybe even the length—of your own life.

Although many people object to being on a special diet, in most cases the meal plan for people with diabetes is more "common sense" than "special". Large amounts of sugar, fats, and salt aren't good for anyone. For the most part, people with diabetes can enjoy a wide variety of nutritious and tasty dishes.

Caring for your own health along with the other person's may also be a way for the two of you to get closer. You might exercise, bike, take long walks, try new recipes, or go to a support group together.

You can make it a team effort to discover new, healthy ways to eat, and, in the case of someone with type 2, to lose weight. You may discover benefits you never thought possible.

What About Your Feelings?

There are times when a situation will trigger feelings of anger, fear, or sadness in you.

It's important to deal with such feelings openly, not bottle them up inside. This may be difficult, especially if there is a family history of sweeping problems under the rug. Remember, your feelings are as valid and important as those of the person with the diabetes.

Holding your feelings in can cause misplaced anger to surface later, when it is inappropriate. The tension produced by holding on to negative feelings might even cause physical symptoms in you.

If the family member with diabetes is doing something that makes you angry, know that your anger is valid. If you are annoyed because they are eating cake and having frequent insulin reactions and don't seem to be testing enough, speak up and make your feelings known.

"Protecting" someone else from the way you feel helps neither of you. Although expressing how you feel may not change the disturbing behavior, he or she will know how much that behavior troubles you.

If you cannot resolve the issues within the family, seek outside professional help. Remember, other people have been there before.

Another emotion you're likely to feel is guilt. It's hard not to feel guilty when you are "allowed" to eat things someone else is not. It's difficult not to feel guilty when you see someone else doing blood tests or taking an injection when you don't have to because your pancreas provides enough insulin for your body.

Of course, it's important not to flaunt this. It's also important not to let the other person feel he or she is making your life miserable because you feel guilty. You can enjoy foods you choose to eat that are not on the other's meal plan.

It's not guilt that helps either of you. It's your understanding of the other person's struggle with a disease that requires daily attention.

You Need Support, Too

You may sometimes feel stressed out from the demands placed on you. This can be especially true when the diabetes causes unstable blood sugars in the other person.

Take care of your stress. Pay attention to your own feelings.

When you feel uncomfortable, when you notice symptoms of anxiety such as a racing heart, nervousness or sweating, stop and take a few deep breaths. Try to figure out what is causing these symptoms. They are signals to you to stop and check in with your body. Failure to do so can result in fear or bottled up anger that is out of proportion to its immediate cause.

The moment you feel that way, it's a good time for you to take a "time out." Maybe some quiet time alone is in order or a call to a friend. Some people keep journals, writing down their feelings to help clarify them and give them a release in writing. Others watch a funny movie, read a book, listen to music. All these can help clear your perspective. The important thing is—take care of you, too.

Sharing feelings with others is often crucial for maintaining a level head in dealing with any chronic illness. Admitting you need help is a sign of strength.

Sometimes even a dear friend cannot sympathize with your problem, however, because he or she hasn't experienced it personally.

There are professional counselors who are trained in chronic disease coping skills. Contact your local affiliate of the American Diabetes Association for information on such programs. Ask doctors, nurses, and diabetes educators where there are such groups in your area.

Many people take comfort in faith. It needn't be an orthodox religion, but simply a higher power concept. For some people, letting go a bit, asking for spiritual help when they are overwhelmed can sometimes ease the burden.

And don't forget humor. It can help diffuse some of the heaviness imposed by dealing with a chronic disease. Laughter helps lighten our load; it relaxes us.

Even if you can't find humor in the midst of a negative situation, you may find yourself laughing later, when you look back on it. One caution: Humor must be gentle and appropriate. Ridicule and teasing that make someone feel singled out obviously do more harm than good.

Keep a good attitude. Be optimistic. When things go wrong, talk together and decide what you'll do differently next time.

Flexibility is a key asset in dealing with diabetes. A sudden episode of hypoglycemia (low blood sugar) or an unexpected hospitalization can cause a sudden change in plans.

Be ready to accept such changes as graciously as possible. The other person is probably feeling bad enough about upsetting arrangements, and the best way you can help is by reassuring them that things will work out. Help them understand that they are more important to you than seeing a movie or going to a party.

Besides being flexible, it's good to have a back-up system for emergencies. Arrange in advance to have a neighbor or friend who can help with what you need— maybe transportation to the hospital, or emotional support for you.

If you do have to go to the hospital, try to have someone meet you there. The person with diabetes will be taken care of by the medical professionals. But a hospital emergency room is a lonely place for you if there is no one to calm your fears.

Finally, don't strive for perfection in your role as a support person. Work for balance. If you check in daily with yourself, you'll know what that balance is.

If there are times you are just not able to give support because your own emotional "well" is dry, be easy on yourself. When you take some time out to nurture yourself, you will come back fresh and restored.

When Your Spouse Has Diabetes

Being married to someone with diabetes can be challenging. Your reactions can significantly influence how well your spouse handles his or her disease.

Having diabetes evokes many emotions. It is not unusual for someone to feel angry or resentful at the unfairness of the situation and wonder, "Why me?"

Someone with diabetes may also feel frustrated and discouraged when he or she finds that it's not always possible to maintain good diabetes control, even by sticking to a recommended self-care plan. Those with diabetes are often concerned about possible long-term complications.

Just knowing the disease is incurable, at least for now, can bring sadness and despair.

As the spouse, you may share some of these feelings. Yet, you have your own emotions, too.

You may have a sense of helplessness in not being able to "rescue" your mate. You may feel neglected if health care providers have not included you in discussions. Even if you are included, you may feel uncertain about your role in the diabetes management.

It's important for both you and your spouse to acknowledge that these feelings exist and to share them honestly. Communicating rather than denying or suppressing your feelings may help bring you closer.

There are a number of ways you might help your mate follow a self-care plan. Agreeing to eat the foods listed in the meal plan and exercising together are good examples. To give your spouse a break from routine and to communicate your desire to be supportive, you might administer his or her insulin, or do the blood glucose testing occasionally.

Couples who are thinking of starting a family have special concerns and need to discuss their feelings about diabetes and children with each other.

Because there are certain hereditary factors in diabetes, you may be concerned about the prospect of having a child who has a greater than average chance of developing the disease. Genetic counseling may help address this question.

Couples, where the wife has diabetes, may wonder about the demands of tight control during pregnancy, possible complications, as well as extra medical costs. Before making a final decision, it's wise for both of you to talk to a physician. The important point is that you are both involved in gathering and evaluating information and making your decision together.

Your sexual relationship is another aspect of marriage that might be affected. Both men and women can become irritable, unusually fatigued, and lose interest in sex if diabetes is not adequately controlled.

It's helpful to recognize that it is the diabetes, not a problem in your relationship, that has brought the lack of sexual responsiveness. You can give support by expressing your understanding, and accepting the need to postpone lovemaking until your partner has improved diabetes control.

Reduced sexual performance is a common long-term complication of diabetes, particularly in men, although not exclusively. If the husband becomes impotent, the wife can help him explore various treatment options.

If this causes problems, both can seek ways of maintaining a satisfying sexual relationship without intercourse. It might help for both partners to see a qualified sex therapist.

Although you do not have diabetes, you might find that you are more committed to good control than your spouse who does have the disease. It can be frustrating and worrisome to live with someone who makes little effort to eat appropriately, monitor blood sugar levels, and exercise regularly.

Suggestions for Giving Support

* Get an education in diabetes care.
* Be supportive, but not a caretaker.
* Help someone you love to keep to the rules, not break them.
* Lend a sympathetic ear.
* Stay flexible.
* Plan for emergencies.
* Make sure others know how to recognize and care for low blood sugars.
* Keep an optimistic, positive attitude.
* Remember that humor can help you both through tough situations.
* Know that your own feelings are valid and that they count.
* Don't strive for perfection in yourself; work for balance in your life.

It's important to remember that the person with diabetes is ultimately responsible for his or her own care. Although you can be a positive influence, neither you nor anyone else can make your partner take good care of himself or herself. Pleading or nagging often makes matters worse. It is appropriate to express your concern, but remember to focus on how you feel about your spouse's behavior. Take responsibility for your feelings and not how your spouse handles his or her diabetes.

—Robert B. Hanks, MA, CRC, CDE

Bonnie Murray *has been involved in intensive care and home care and occupational health nursing. She is on the Johns Hopkins Diabetes Center Council and is active in the Johns Hopkins Insulin Pump Club. She is also the wife of a man with insulin-dependent diabetes.* **Robert Hanks** *is a Licensed Counselor at Providence Hospital in Mobile, Alabama.*

Self-Care Titles

ADA Complete Guide to Diabetes
Every area of self-care is covered in this ultimate diabetes reference for your home.
Hardcover. #CSMCGD
Nonmember: $29.95/ADA Member: $23.95

101 Tips for Staying Healthy With Diabetes
Get the inside track on the latest tips, techniques, and strategies for preventing and treating diabetes complications.
Softcover. #CSMFSH
Nonmember: $12.50/ADA Member: $9.95

How to Get Great Diabetes Care
Informs you of the importance of seeking medical attention that meets the ADA Standards of Care.
Softcover. #CSMHGGDC
Nonmember: $11.95/ADA Member: $9.55

Sweet Kids: How to Balance Diabetes Control & Good Nutrition with Family Peace
This new guide addresses behavioral and developmental issues of nutrition management.
Softcover. #CSMSK
Nonmember: $14.95/ADA Member: $11.95

Reflections on Diabetes
A collection of stories written by people who have learned from the experience of living with the disease.
Softcover. #CSMROD
Nonmember: $9.95/ADA Member: $7.95

Cookbooks

How To Cook for People with Diabetes
#CCBCFPD
Nonmember: $11.95/ADA Member: $9.55

Southern-Style Diabetic Cooking
#CCBSSDC
Nonmember: $11.95/ADA Member: $9.55

Flavorful Seasons Cookbook
#CCBFS
Nonmember: $16.95/ADA Member: $13.55

World-Class Diabetic Cooking
#CCBWCC
Nonmember: $12.95/ADA Member: $11.65

Magic Menus
#CCBMM
Nonmember: $14.95/ADA Member: $11.95

Diabetic Meals in 30 Minutes—Or Less!
#CCBDM
Nonmember: $11.95/ADA Member: $9.55

Diabetes Meal Planning Made Easy
#CCBMP
Nonmember: $14.95/ADA Member: $11.95

To order call:
1-800-ADA-ORDER (232-6733)

For membership information call:
1-800-DIABETES (342-2383)